The Alexander Technique

A Skill for Life

Pedro de Alcantara

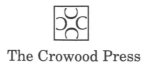

The Crowood Press

First published in 1999 by
The Crowood Press Ltd
Ramsbury, Marlborough
Wiltshire SN8 2HR

www.crowood.com

This impression 2004

British Library Cataloguing-in-Publication Data
A catalogue record for this book is available from the British Library.

ISBN 1 86126 286 8

Typefaces used: Galliard and Franklin Gothic.

Typeset and designed by
D & N Publishing
Lambourn Woodlands, Hungerford, Berkshire.

Printed and bound in Great Britain by CPI Bath.

Photo Credits and Acknowledgements
Drawings ©Alexis Niki, by permission, with warmest thanks. Photographs of F. M. Alexander ©1999 The Society of Teachers of the Alexander Technique. Cheetah: ©Fritz Polking/Agence Jacana, by permission. Baseball players: ©Frank Gunn/AP, by permission. Caroline: courtesy of Catherine de Chevilly, with warm thanks. Iolane Luahine: ©Topgalant Publishing Co., with warm thanks to Sandra Kwock-Silve. 'The World is a Harmony of Tensions': ©Hassan Massoudy/Editions du Désastre, by kind permission of the artist, with warm thanks. 'Jumping over a boy's back': from *Animal Locomotion* by Eadweard Muybridge, ©Dover Publications, Inc., by kind permission. Boy in a deep monkey: with warm thanks to Michelle and Bernard. Girl lunging: courtesy of Brigitte Cavadias, with warm thanks. Boy at the beach: courtesy of Joelle Schneider, with warm thanks. Ivo playing soccer, and at the end of the book: courtesy of Magdalena Pasikowska, with warm thanks to Jörg Schnass. Stills from "Min Agl Hobbi" and "Risalat Gharam": ©Institut du Monde Arabe, by kind permission of Films Regent. Aung San Suu Kyi: ©Tom Pilston/*The Independent*, by permission, with thanks and much affection to Marjorie Hodge. Artur Rubinstein: ©Lotte Meitner-Graf, courtesy of the Rubinstein family. Annie, aged six: courtesy of Richard Beavitt and Annie Robinson, with warm thanks. Despite his best efforts, the author was unable to contact the copyright holders of the photos of Alfred Cortot and Yukiyoshi Sagawa.

Excerpt from *World of Wonders* by Robertson Davies (Penguin Books, 1977), published in *The Deptford Trilogy* (Penguin Books, 1983), copyright ©Robertson Davies, 1975. Reproduced by permission of Penguin Books Ltd. and Pendragon Ink.

Portions of Phyllis Richmond's essay, *The Actor and the Character*, appeared originally in *Curiosity Recaptured*, edited by Jerry Sontag (San Francisco: Mornum Time Press, 1996).

Contents

Acknowledgements

In the summer of 1994 I received an invitation from Editions Dangles, a French publishing house, to write an introductory book on the Alexander Technique for their catalogue. I owe this invitation to my colleague Annie Moteï, and the existence of my French book, *La Technique Alexander: Principes et Pratique*, to the perseverance of the late Jean-Yves Anstet-Dangles, who prodded me along – no, who *threatened* me – when I started doubting that I could write a book in French. Since *The Alexander Technique* is a younger brother to *Principes et Pratique*, I owe its existence too to Annie and Monsieur Anstet-Dangles.

Several of my pupils and friends, including April Cowan, Katherine Fredrickson, Melanie Meunier and Edward Lamont, read excerpts from my manuscript and offered invaluable comments. I have received notarized statements from most of them swearing that they are not responsible for my book's glaring defects. My wonderfully literate friend Claire de Obaldia midwifed both the French and English versions of this book; without her intervention I would have given a collective heart attack to the members of the Académie Française. (Come to think of it, that would not be such a bad thing.)

My friend Alexis Niki has played a pivotal role, supplying drawings for the book, a testimonial about her Alexander experiences, and her unwavering support for my work. I wish to thank Jean O. M. Fisher for putting me in touch with The Crowood Press. Mr Fisher's company, Mouritz, publishes some of the finest books about the Alexander Technique.

When I set out to write this book, I had the clever idea of asking my pupils and my fellow Alexander teachers to write most of it for me; their generous contributions have become the backbone of the book. To Alexis, Alison, Edward, Geneviève and Liz, and to Malcolm Balk, Patricia Boulay, Catherine de Chevilly and Phyllis Richmond I wish to dedicate *The Alexander Technique*.

Paris, 30 January 1999

Introduction

'My back is hurting me, I think my bed is too soft.'

'My son is so stubborn, he never obeys me.'

'You breathe badly; you should do some breathing exercises. Go on, take a deep breath.'

'That man is irritating.'

'My shoulders are tight.'

'I have scoliosis.'

'Grandma is getting older; it is natural for her back to become a bit round.'

'Life in a big city is so stressful, I wish I could move to the country.'

'I hate my body.'

'I love my body.'

'That is just the way I am, there is nothing I can do about it.'

'He is so intelligent, what a pity he beats his wife.'

'Relax.'

'Sit straight.'

'Swimming is the best exercise.'

'My mother-in-law is horribly unpleasant. I detest her.'

'I try my hardest, but I lack willpower.'

'Stop crying, for heaven's sake!'

You have undoubtedly used similar phrases, and heard them used: by a friend, in school, at the gym, at the doctor's surgery. Such phrases describe a situation, a person's character, or an attitude. Many of the phrases evoke a problem; some of them point to a solution too. In certain phrases, the problem is explicit, while the solution is implicit; sometimes it is the other way around. Each phrase is based on objective observations and highlights a fact, a reality or a truth.

It is true that life in the country is easier than life in a big city. It is true that old people are naturally round-backed. It is true that a soft bed can cause back trouble. It is true that everybody should sit up straight. It is true that deep breathing is good for you.

Observations, thoughts, words, and actions are all intimately connected. People observe this or that fact – a reality or truth – and draw conclusions from their observations, such as 'x' causes 'y'. They then act upon those conclusions:

'My mother-in-law is mean. Everybody knows that. Well, I have to defend myself, and the only way with her is to be as mean as she is.'

'My back is hurting me. My bed is obviously too soft, so I am going to buy a firm mattress.'

'My shoulders are tight. That is because I am under a lot of stress at work. I need a good massage.'

In the last example, the diagnosis includes a description of symptoms ('shoulders are tight'), an analysis of their cause ('stress'), and a proposed remedy ('a massage'). Now it is possible to draw a general principle. For each problem there is a corresponding description, an analysis, and a solution. Living means facing problems, analysing and understanding them, and finding solutions for them. This may be done consciously or subconsciously, using intuition, reason, imagination, intellect, and other faculties; however it is done, everyone does it constantly.

But what if a problem is misunderstood? What if the description of a problem is based on false perceptions, and the analysis on flawed assumptions? What if the remedy aggravates the problem? This book will show how, in fact, the great majority of people's perceptions, suppositions, descriptions, analyses, diagnoses, and solutions are incorrect.

When someone says, 'My shoulders are tight', this is not exactly true. It would be more accurate – and ultimately more useful – to say, 'I am tightening my shoulders.' Similarly, when people complain about back pain, it is *they* who are hurting their backs, not their backs that are hurting *them*.

'My work is a lot of stress.' Four people in the same stressful situation will reaction in four different, if not opposing, ways. For example, in a typical office after the boss announces a new development, Peter becomes mute, Jean worries, Harry gets to work, while Anna rings her sister to gossip and laugh for a minute. Stress is not a stimulus, but a reaction to it, whether it is a situation, a person, or an idea. (The imagination is the source of many troubles.) Peter and Jean react in a manner that is neither constructive nor practical, and are therefore likely to consider themselves to be 'under stress'. Anna and Harry react differently, and would probably talk differently about the situation as well.

'I need a good massage.' At the end of an hour under the massage practitioner's hands, you feel deliciously relaxed. Next morning, you go back to work to find that your boss is still alive and kicking. How do you deal with that?

Some people react to certain situations by contracting their shoulders. A massage may help you feel good temporarily, but it will not alter the root cause of your tensions, which are your own reactions to the world around you. Indeed, you will not succeed in loosening your shoulders and, most importantly, in keeping them loose, until you change the way you react. Alexander would describe this as the way you 'use yourself'.

'Sit straight.' This simple command reflects a world of assumptions. There is a good position that you must hold, which is, of course, straight. It implies a certain relationship between the body and the will, and a course of action that flows from their interaction. If you have a physical problem ('bad posture'), take care of it by doing something ('sit straight'). All you have to do is apply your will to it. If you cannot manage to sit straight, it is because your will is weak.

Frederick Matthias Alexander – actor and pedagogue, savant and visionary, rogue extraordinaire – says, first and foremost, that body and mind are inseparable. We used to think of the body as a car, and the mind as its driver. Today, we compare the body with a computer, and the mind with a programmer. Both metaphors are wrong. For, in human beings, the thing controlled, the force that controls it, and the control itself are one. Therefore, the mind cannot be master of the body; rather, the mind is the body, and the body is the mind. Regardless of the problem ('bad posture'), a will that is weak or insufficient cannot be the cause of the problem. Neither can strength of will be a solution in itself, as long as problem and solution both imply a separation between the body and the mind. (*See* especially Chapter 1.)

On the subject of 'sitting straight', Alexander says that there are no good positions, but only directions, which make a given position healthy or unhealthy. The idea is not to seek a position ('sitting straight'), but a direction ('upwards', for example). He would add that a problem cannot be solved by doing the right thing, but by stopping doing the wrong one.

When you 'sit straight', you are trying to do the right thing, but this is sure to lead to failure, as everyone who has ever tried to improve his or her posture would testify. (Chapter 2 discusses posture, while Chapter 6 offers a testimonial from a woman who once laboured under the notion that her posture was bad and her will weak.) Instead of sitting straight (something that you *do*), it would be better to stop slumping (something that you *stop doing*). Stop doing what is wrong, and the right thing will do itself. A source of great revelation and equally great difficulty, this principle – which Alexander named 'Inhibition', thereby perplexing the uninitiated – is the cornerstone of the Alexander Technique. (Inhibition and its counterpart, direction, are discussed in Chapter 3.)

Alexander would also recommend that you do not try to change the habits of someone else – a member of your family, a colleague at work, a close friend – by nagging, and giving instructions such as 'sit up straight', 'relax', 'calm down', or 'use your brain'. All your relationships start with the way you present yourself to others, and you should therefore aim to become a living model of that which you wish to see in others. This golden rule, made all the more resplendent by your *non-doing*, is bound to change the dynamics of your relationships, thereby indirectly affecting the behaviour of the people around you. (Find out the truth about your mother-in-law in Chapter 5.)

The fundamental unity of every human being; our habits, behaviours, suppositions, and judgements; the difference between 'normal' and 'natural'; ergonomics and physiotherapy; posture, attitude, movement, tension and relaxation, inhibition and direction; social and professional relationships, sports and exercise, music, theatre, and dance: in sum, health and well-being are the objects of this study. My aim is to convince you that your problems are not what you think they are, and to propose simple and efficient solutions which bear witness to the genius of a great man: Frederick Matthias Alexander.

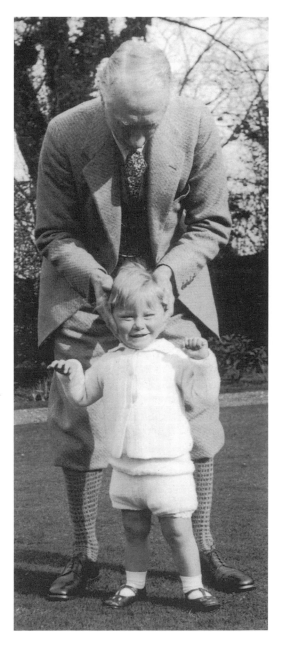

CHAPTER 1
First Principles

A MISDIAGNOSED PROBLEM

To understand the principles of the Alexander Technique, it is useful to look back at what F. M. Alexander himself set out to do. He described his journey in detail in the first chapter of *The Use of the Self*, the third of his four books. The ethologist Nikolaas Tinbergen, winner of the 1973 Nobel Prize for Physiology or Medicine, dedicated part of his Nobel oration to Alexander and his work. Alexander's story, Tinbergen wrote, 'of perceptiveness, of intelligence, and of persistence, shown by a man without medical training, is one of the true epics of medical research and practice'.[1]

Frederick Matthias Alexander was born in 1869 in Tasmania, off the south coast of Australia. A young man of promise, he hoped to pursue a career as a professional actor. His great passion was Shakespeare, which he declaimed in the dramatic recitals that were popular at the time. Despite his acting talent, his career was threatened by a recurring vocal problem – on stage, he tended to become hoarse, sometimes even losing his voice. Alexander sought medical advice and was told to rest his voice. While his voice was protected as long as he refrained from using it, the hoarseness returned as soon as he began to work on the stage again. He was then advised to undergo surgery, the diagnosis being that his uvula was too long.

Resting the voice is sensible if it is over-used. An operation is equally sensible if there is a structural problem somewhere in the vocal mechanism. However, Alexander suspected that his vocal problems were due neither to his over-using his voice, nor to a defect of his vocal mechanism itself. Rather, he reasoned that the source of his difficulties was actually the way in which he used his voice.

This may seem obvious to the modern reader, but in turn-of-the-century Australia most people would either have persisted with the rest cure or agreed to undergo surgery, without daring to contradict the view of a doctor. Alexander's outlook was well ahead of his time.

Second, even today many people are still reluctant to accept that the cause of their problems is something that they do to themselves. In this instance, medicine plays a role, as it did a century ago. One example is carpal tunnel syndrome, a painful and possibly disabling condition that affects musicians, keyboard operators, and other people in various occupations and circumstances. When diagnosing carpal tunnel syndrome, doctors speak of over-use of the wrist, and prescribe rest. If rest fails, medicine offers the choice of surgery or injections of cortisone. Cortisone acts temporarily upon a symptom of the disease, namely the pain, and it may have dangerous side-effects too. Surgery is not free from risk and does not offer guaranteed results. In any case, doctors' current understanding of disease and cure shows that Alexander's insight – original and revolutionary as it was a hundred years ago – today remains as pertinent as ever. Even more 'modern' solutions to carpal tunnel syndrome – physiotherapy, in the form of exercises for the wrist, and ergonomics, which alters the work environment – fail to diagnose and treat the problem adequately.

THE UNITY OF BEING

To have a better appreciation of Alexander's understanding of the cause and effect involved in his voice loss, it is useful to read his own words:

> When I began my investigation, I, in common with most people, conceived of 'body' and 'mind' as separate parts of the same organism, and consequently believed that human ills, difficulties, and shortcomings could be classified as either 'mental' or 'physical' and dealt with on specifically 'mental' or specifically 'physical' lines.

Alexander went on to say that he soon abandoned this point of view, stating that his experiences led him to believe that 'it is impossible to separate "mental" and "physical" processes in any form of human activity.'[2]

In its theory and its practice, the Technique highlights the ever-present connection that exists between body and mind – indeed, their very inseparability. Alexander was keenly aware of the links between the way we think and the way we speak, and he avoided – in his teaching as well as in his writings – using terms such as 'body mechanics' or 'mental complexes'. Instead, he referred to the human psycho-physical organism in its entirety as 'the self', and spoke of how this 'self' 'reacts' and 'functions'.

The term 'self', as employed by Alexander, does not have the connotations that are now attributed to it by psychoanalysts (as in the opposition between 'self' and 'other', for instance). Rather, it is a simple way of referring to the whole person at once. Even to speak of body, mind, and spirit working together implies some separateness between the parts. This has important practical consequences. If you think that you are composed of separate parts, you are likely to conceive of the source of some difficulty or shortcoming as one of those parts and to seek solutions specific to each part, and in isolation from the workings of the whole.

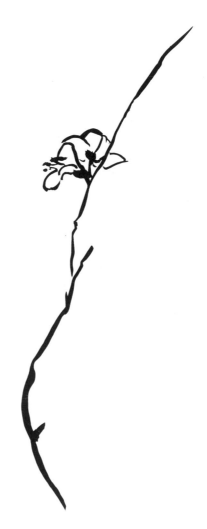

Deeply rooted, the plant grows ever upwards.

Taking lessons in the Technique will give you a practical understanding of your wholeness, which may escape you if you limit your study to reading about the subject. However, all students of the Technique can get off to a good start by cultivating the habit of thinking and speaking not of the way they use their bodies, but of the way they use themselves.

Grasping the meaning of 'the self' may be made easier by considering an example of 'the use of the self'. Imagine yourself in a concrete situation – walking down the street, playing tennis, making love. In any of these, every part of your being is present, whether the part plays a passive role or an active one. The tennis player cannot lift a racket (thereby making a physical gesture) without issuing a command from the brain to the muscles via the nerves (thereby engaging the mind). Body and mind act together, at once, always, whether they do so efficiently or not. Similarly, when you make love, every fibre of your being plays a role. The intense physical pleasure of making love has equally intense psychological, emotional and intellectual counterparts. Perhaps you are unaware of the intimate connection between body and mind as you make love; still, your lack of awareness does not deny the existence of the connection. Becoming aware of the wholeness of your acts will reinforce their beauty and intensity, whether you are making love, playing tennis, singing a lullaby to a child, or eating an ice-cream.

The integrity of your being means that your whole body, from head to toe, plays a role in every activity. Different parts play different roles – some roles are more passive, others are more active, some are very important, and others are less so. For the integrated lover, the entire body is erogenous; for the integrated sportsman or musician, the entire body is an instrument. Indeed, in all human endeavour, every body part plays a role, at all times.

Alexander's vocal troubles were the root of his approach to the Technique. The cause of his hoarseness on stage was not misuse of his voice, but rather the way he co-ordinated himself as he spoke. In *The Use of the Self* he wrote that, as he declaimed, he pulled his head back and down, depressed his larynx, shortened his torso, and tensed his legs and feet. In order to eliminate his vocal problem, then, it was not enough for Alexander to change the use of his voice; he had to change the co-ordination of his whole being – that is, the way he used himself.

USE AND FUNCTIONING

The way you use yourself affects every aspect of your functioning, including your manner of speech and the timbre of your voice; your breathing, digestion, and circulation; your psychomotor skills and reactions to stress; your interpersonal relationships, emotions, and sexuality. The relationship between use and functioning is undoubtedly the most practical of Alexander's discoveries. If you wish to improve any aspect of your functioning, you must improve your use. If you use your whole self well, every one of your activities will contribute to your greater well-being. If you use yourself badly, all that you do will harm your health. In Chapter 2, the characteristics of good use of the self are described. In subsequent chapters, the relationship between use and emotions, general health, dietary habits, sports and exercise, and other areas of your life are discussed. However, this is a good point at which to attempt a definition of 'the use of the self'.

The way you use yourself is the way you react, with your entire being, in every situation of your life. In some situations you react well, healthily, with efficiency, intelligence, and elegance. In other situations, you react less well. Whether you react well or badly, your whole being is present in all your reactions, and your body – from head to toe – is always inseparable from the thinking that animates it. 'Talk about a man's individuality and character,' Alexander liked saying. 'It's the way he uses himself.'[3]

PHYSIOTHERAPY AND ERGONOMICS

In comparing modern medicine with the approaches that were common in Alexander's time, I mentioned physiotherapy and ergonomics as two sciences that offer new solutions to old health problems. As they are generally practised today, both tend to overlook the fundamental indivisibility of the human being – the concept on which Alexander built his entire work.

Physiotherapy

Faced with a patient who suffers from carpal tunnel syndrome, for example, a physiotherapist may prescribe a series of wrist and hand exercises. Nevertheless, the real cause of the syndrome is not over-use of the wrist, or even its misuse. Rather, the badly used wrist is a symptom of the patient's misuse of his or her whole self. This misuse is inextricably linked to a series of perceptions, attitudes, and beliefs. If the sufferer performs wrist exercises without having changed the attitudes that animate his or her gestures, the situation may well be aggravated instead of alleviated. Further, no exercise is beneficial in itself; its capacity to do good depends upon the way in which it is practised. Because of faulty sensory awareness (*see* later in this chapter), a patient or student risks carrying out well-designed exercises ineptly, despite his or her best intentions. A clever exercise ineptly performed can often be more harmful than beneficial.

Ergonomics

The young science of ergonomics has brought interesting innovations into many fields, including furniture and machinery design and the organization of work routines. Nevertheless, some of its precepts must be considered with circumspection, as received wisdom is sometimes wrong. For instance, there is a widely accepted notion that a very firm mattress is good for the back, yet a mattress that is too firm will not follow the natural curves of the human body. Many people are uncomfortable in bed, but persist in the belief that their over-hard mattress is good for their back.

Since human beings are so different from each other, morphologically as well as psychologically, it is impossible to find a universal solution to every postural difficulty. An armchair may be perfectly suitable for one person and quite awkward for another. More importantly, what is comfortable is not necessarily healthy. Many pieces of furniture are designed to accommodate not the *ideal* use of the self, but rather the *habitual* use. Many people collapse into their armchairs and sofas; although they are twisting and compacting their bodies, they will tell you that they feel very comfortable indeed. Inversely, some chairs and sofas are designed to direct your body into a well-balanced state. If the seated person is not used to such a state, however, he or she may well find these pieces of furniture uncomfortable.

Some pieces of furniture make it more or less easy for you to direct your use, while others make it more or less difficult. However, no piece of furniture can *force* you to assume a naturally healthy position; indeed, that would be a contradiction in terms. In sum, the usefulness of ergonomics will always be limited by a large number of factors: the enormous differences from person to person; the gap between what is comfortable and what is healthy; and, above all, the difficulty of benefiting from a well-

11

designed and well-constructed piece of furniture if you lack the necessary ability to direct yourself.

It is certainly cost-effective for you to deepen your knowledge of the principles of good use before replacing your furniture, at work or at home.

THE CAUSES OF MISUSE

Alexander equated a person's individuality and character with the way he or she uses the self. He might well have said that a person's character is the way he or she *mis*uses the self, for most people misuse themselves most of the time, thereby causing themselves much discomfort, and even disease and disability.

What causes misuse? The answer to this simple question again attests to Alexander's genius. Most people would readily blame education, civilization, modern life, stress, religion, the lack of religion, family life, other people. Alexander believed otherwise, recognizing that the problem lies not in what is done to the individual, but in what the individual does to himself. Faced with the constant stimulation of life, you can react healthily (using the best means any situation requires of you), or unhealthily (neglecting the means whereby your end may be achieved, and going straight for your end regardless of the price you may have to pay). The final cause of misuse, in Alexander's view, is the universal habit of 'end-gaining'.

Imagine a father and his child. The child is upset and crying. The father's single wish is for the child to stop crying. Yet, rather than finding out why she is upset and consoling her, he yells at her to stop crying, which only makes her cry harder. By end-gaining – that is, by going directly to his desired end while disregarding the best means of getting there – the father makes a bad situation worse, both for the child and for himself.

It would be easy to make a list of hundreds of instances of end-gaining in all spheres of human activity. End-gaining is so prevalent and insidious that most people do not realize that they, and others, are doing it all the time. Business, politics, medicine, art, daily life, and personal relationships are all subject to the damages of end-gaining thought and behaviour. Examples of this will be found throughout this book.

End-gaining causes misuse, and misuse causes poor functioning. To improve your functioning, you need to stop misusing yourself; to stop misusing yourself, you need to stop end-gaining. This points to another of Alexander's brilliant insights. To change the way you use yourself, the important thing is not what you *do*, but what you *stop doing* and what you prevent yourself from doing. This is the cornerstone of the Alexander Technique, referred to in our technical vocabulary as 'inhibition' (with a different definition from that of the psychologists). Alexandrian inhibition does not mean repressing or suppressing your feelings, but, rather, refraining from reacting in a habitual, unreasoned, and harmful manner. To inhibit is to stop end-gaining. When you end-gain, you do too much too soon; when you inhibit, you stop doing. Inhibition (or *non-doing*) sets the Technique apart from the majority of other approaches to problem-solving, which are normally based on trying to do the right thing. Inhibition is discussed at length in Chapter 3.

THE PRIMARY CONTROL

When Alexander made his series of linked discoveries, he concluded that direct control of any aspect of human functioning – breathing, digestion, or the use of a specific muscle, for instance – is, depending on the case, unnecessary, possibly harmful, or just plain impossible. But if we are not to control the

The Head Leads, the Body Follows

The cheetah demonstrates to perfection the workings of the Primary Control, which all vertebrates share. In brief, the orientation of the head in relation to the body establishes the co-ordination of the whole body. Note that 'orientation' and 'position' are two different matters; the cheetah may place its head in an infinite number of quickly changing positions, but it orients it in a nearly unvarying direction, forward and up away from the body. Even when it turns its head back and down in space, the cheetah never allows the weight of its head to contract its neck or shorten its spine.

In this photo, the cheetah's head is not straight in relation to the body, showing that symmetry of position need not be a concern of well co-ordinated animals, be they feline or human. In other words, to hold your head straight will not improve your co-ordination; but to direct it in a supple and dynamic manner certainly will.

When you first attempt to direct your Primary Control consciously, you are likely to over-tense your neck; while attempting to relax your neck, you are likely to over-slacken your spine. The cheetah's movements are characterized by well-distributed tension, not relaxation. Its limbs are all powerfully connected to its head and spine; in this photo, this is evident particularly in the line that runs from the head to the end of the right front paw.

To appreciate the importance of the Primary Control, imagine what would happen if, while hunting, the cheetah contracted its head backwards into the spine: Dinner would escape, and the species would be doomed.

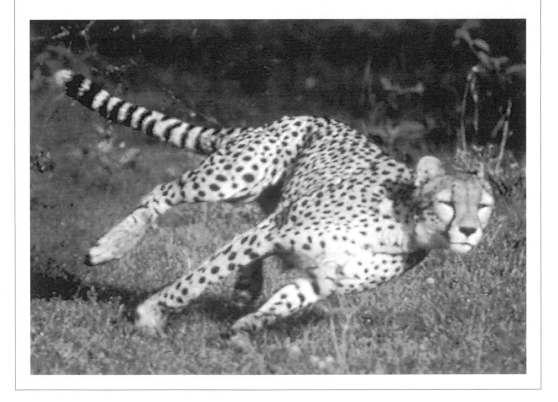

Two Minnesota Twins: Alex Ochoa, an out-fielder, and Todd Walker, the second baseman as shown below. Compare these athletes with each other, and both with the cheetah. Ochoa, behind Walker, holds himself asymmetrically; yet, since his head remains beautifully directed, his co-ordination does not suffer from the asymmetry. In his case, the neck belongs to the spine, not to the head; the shoulders belong to the back, not to the arms; and the pelvis belongs to the back, not to the legs. The only apparent flaw in his stance is the over-tense right hand.

The impression we have from looking at Walker, though, is that he leads with his chest when he leaps forwards and upwards; by sheer inertia, his head gets thrown back. The down-ward pull of his head breaks the line between neck and spine, causing his back to shorten and narrow and his pelvis to tilt too far backwards – in all, a striking illustration of how the misdi-rected Primary Control affects the co-ordination of the whole body.

Had Walker led with his head, not his chest, he would have been able to afford an asymmetrical position of his head in relation to the body, like Ochoa and the cheetah. As it was, dinner escaped: Walker bobbled the pop fly and the Toronto Blue Jays beat the Twins, 6–0.

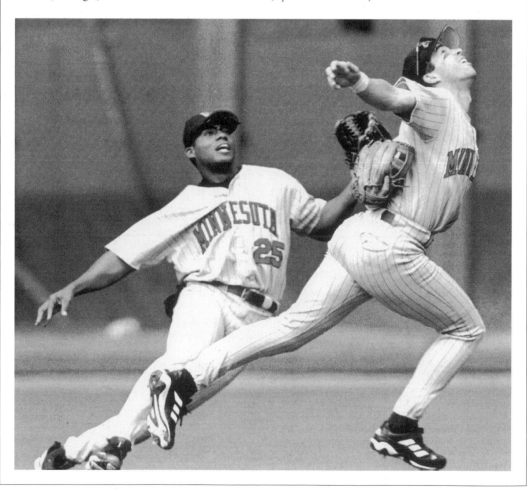

functioning of our organisms, how can we change and grow, and achieve good health and well-being?

Alexander observed that in all human beings – and, indeed, in all vertebrates – there exists an ever-changing, dynamic relationship between the head, the neck, and the back. He called it the Primary Control, and demonstrated that the way you use your Primary Control determines your total co-ordination directly, and your functioning indirectly. In other words, the better you use your Primary Control, the better your total co-ordination will be; and the better your co-ordination, the better your functioning. Inversely, if you misuse your Primary Control, you are likely to suffer a deterioration in your co-ordination, and, consequently, in your health and well-being.

The Primary Control is not synonymous with a single position. Given the right co-ordinative conditions, all positions of the head and neck can be healthy. Someone such as Fred Astaire – a fine example of elegance, suppleness, and well-directed strength – could put his head in any position without harming himself. In the absence of the right co-ordinative conditions – which, for example, made Astaire a great dancer – most positions of the head and neck are unhealthy, some more so than others. For example, pulling the head back and down is particularly harmful, as the weight of the head then bears down upon the neck and spine, shortening and narrowing the whole back.

A particular position – of the head, of a limb, of the whole body – becomes 'right' or 'wrong' according to the directions that precede and accompany it. (This proposition will become clearer when directions are discussed later.) If you are well co-ordinated – that is, well directed – you need not concern yourself with positioning your head. However, if you wish to improve your co-ordination, you need to become aware of the positions in which you place your head, so that you are better able to understand the mechanisms by which you co-ordinate your whole self. Once you become aware of how you direct your Primary Control, you can then let go of any concerns about positioning your head and neck.

In human beings of average co-ordination, misuse of the Primary Control is so prevalent that it has become difficult to appreciate the beauty of its workings. Animals, both wild and domesticated, are better models of good co-ordination. When a cat jumps up on to a table, its head leads, and its body follows. When a horse is jumping fences, its whole body is taut with strength and joy, from the head downwards. Its head leads, and its body follows. At all times its spine remains fully stretched, and its head poised strongly on top of the neck. When a bear forages for food, its head leads, and its body follows, even as the bear becomes occasionally upright. When a seagull glides in the wind, its head leads, its body follows. Its whole spine is stretched and in a state of high tonus, and the seagull thus becomes aerodynamic. Indeed, it would be impossible for a bird to fly or to glide if its spine were too relaxed.

Every healthy small child displays the same state of co-ordination and high tonus. It is fascinating to watch a baby learning how to crawl or walk. The way the baby uses her head and neck determines whether her movements are easy and elegant or awkward and laboured. The same applies for the older child learning how to ice-skate or ride a bicycle. Soon, however, most children lose their natural, animal-like poise, through imitation, education, and simple end-gaining.

Once you begin to understand Alexander's theory of the Primary Control, you will see how every adult who displays real composure and freedom uses his or her head, neck, and back like the baby, the child, the cat and the dog, the seagull and the bear. In effect, it is

When Caroline, eighteen months old, leans forwards, her head plays a double role. Before, during, and after her every move, Caroline points her head up away from her body, thereby

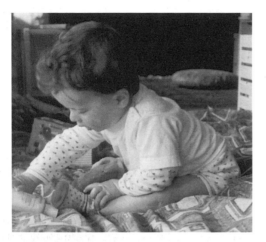

allowing her spine to remain optimally elongated. When she leans forwards in space, Caroline initiates the movement with her head, which carries on allowing the stretch of the spine. In other words, she *points up* to *move forwards*, and in both instances – in the pointing and in the moving – her head leads and her body follows. Her Primary Control works in an entirely instinctive manner, like the cheetah's.

The late Iolani Luahine, a great Hawaiian dancer, also points up to move forwards. Once upon a time she too was eighteen months old, and we can easily suppose that at the time she used her Primary Control in an instinctive manner, similar to Caroline's. Through the conscious application of her kinaesthetic intelligence, she enhanced what was innate and made it *intuitive*, rather than instinctive, thus accomplishing the passage from childhood to mastery.

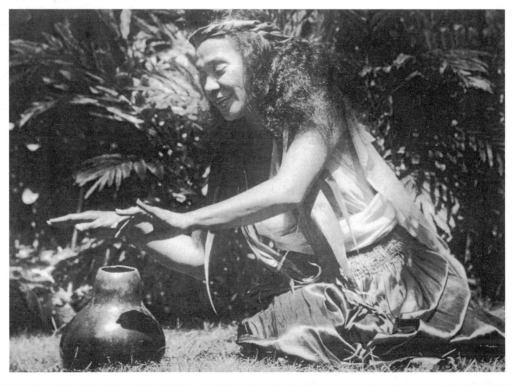

thanks to the poise of the Primary Control that such an adult is able to master himself or herself, and to be well co-ordinated and healthy.

The goal of the Alexander pupil is not to learn how to control the body or its functioning. Instead, the aim is to stop interfering with the natural workings of the head, neck, and back, and to prevent this interference from happening again. Re-directing the head, neck, and back does not entail doing the right thing; it means stopping doing the wrong one. Think again about the cat, the seagull, and the baby. Their good co-ordination, their freedom and well-being are not the result of a conscious muscular effort, but the *absence* of such an effort. When you stop misusing your Primary Control – when you stop doing the wrong things – you allow your organism to assume its optimum state, which is dynamic, vigorous, elastic, and strong.

Let us imagine that you seek an Alexander teacher because you suffer from asthma, or tendonitis, or stage fright. Regardless of your initial motivation to study the Technique, your teacher is likely to avoid working directly on your complaint. Instead, he or she will help you become aware of how you use your Primary Control – or, rather, of how you misuse it. Then you will be helped to stop this misuse and to prevent it from recurring. As a result, your total co-ordination (or the way you use yourself) will improve, thereby mitigating or eliminating the condition for which you sought the teacher in the first place.

The above is an indirect approach. It has many merits, which are discussed throughout this book. It is enough to note here that when you stop misusing your Primary Control, the resulting changes in co-ordination and attitude are all-encompassing and, to a degree, automatic. According to Alexander, 'In cases where the knowledge of how to direct the primary control has led to a change for the better in the manner of the use of the mechanisms throughout the organism, the results of this "conditioning" can safely be left to take their own form'.[4]

Very many people approach an Alexander teacher trying to rid themselves of a single specific complaint – backache or a breathing problem, for instance – and end up improving every facet of their life, *and* ridding themselves of the complaint in the process.

SENSORY AWARENESS AND HABIT

Alexander recognized that there are several obstacles to change. Two of these are interrelated. First, most people are unaware of their uses and misuses. They are unlikely to perceive accurately what they are doing and how they are doing it. For instance, when most people see pictures or videos of themselves, they exclaim, 'This can't be me! I'm not like that!' There is a gap between what they do and what they think they do, and between who they are and who they feel themselves to be. Alexander called this 'faulty sensory awareness', an almost universal phenomenon that plays a fundamental role in the Technique.

We all learn in school that we have five senses: sight, hearing, smell, taste, and touch. Yet we have another sense, of which we are less aware, despite its great importance to our health and well-being. Indeed, being oblivious to this all-important sense is one of the reasons we become unhealthy.

Muscles, joints, and tendons have sense organs called proprioceptors, which send feedback to the nervous system about the position of a body part relative to the rest of the body. Proprioception is the body's sense of itself. Laymen refer to it by the somewhat vague term of 'muscle sense'. The neck muscles are particularly well supplied with proprioceptors. By misusing your head and neck, you cause such distortions to your proprioception that it ceases to be reliable, thereby affecting your sensation of position, movement, balance, tonus, tension, relaxation, effort, and fatigue. A vicious circle then develops: the more you misuse yourself, the less reliable your sensory awareness becomes; and as your sense impressions grow ever more inaccurate, your use deteriorates accordingly. Alexander developed an imaginative and effective way of breaking this vicious circle; this is described in detail in Chapter 4.

Closely intertwined with sensory awareness is a second obstacle to change: habit. The brain tends to place new thoughts and new perceptions in the foreground, and to push old information to the background. We get so used to our gestures, our voices, and our smells, that we end up taking them for granted, and finish by ignoring them. We do not pay attention to what is habitual, in the vain hope of being better able to process and understand what is unfamiliar. This lack of attention leads in time to neglect and distortion. As it turns out, the way we perceive ourselves colours, and often determines, the way we see others. Therefore, by neglecting, ignoring or distorting the information we have about ourselves – by pushing habitual information to the background – we end up misjudging and misunderstanding information that we receive from others and about others. Habit, sensory awareness, and the use we make of ourselves are, then, three distinct but intimately connected manifestations of a single entity.

THE PRINCIPLES OF THE TECHNIQUE

At this point, it is useful to summarize the main principles of the Alexander Technique so far discussed. You will find that all other aspects of the Technique, theoretical as well as practical, follow naturally and logically from these main points.

- To highlight and enhance the fundamental wholeness of a human being, Alexander spoke of 'the self' rather than the body or the mind.
- To highlight and enhance the fundamental dynamism of a human being, Alexander spoke of 'the use of the self' rather than body mechanics, posture, mental states, or mental complexes. The self 'reacts' and 'functions'.
- Alexander demonstrated that the way you use yourself affects all aspects of your functioning. By misusing yourself, you cause a deterioration in the way you function. It follows that, to improve functioning, you must improve the way you use yourself.
- Misuse, in turn, is caused by the universal habit of end-gaining. To improve your use, you need not 'do the right thing', but stop doing the wrong one – that is, stop end-gaining. This is called 'inhibition', and it becomes operational through the use of directions. Remember that you do not inhibit misuse; instead, you inhibit the end-gaining of which misuse is an effect.
- Alexander established that the orientation of the head in relation to the neck, and of both head and neck in relation to the back, determine total co-ordination. He called this relationship the Primary Control. The better you direct your Primary Control, the better your whole co-ordination (and consequently your functioning) will be.
- Faulty sensory awareness and the force of habit are two of the greatest obstacles to change and growth.

(All these principles interact in ways that make it difficult to discuss them separately. As the following chapters focus on each principle, constant references will be made to the other principles. In an introductory discussion of a new subject, repetitions will be inevitable and are, perhaps, desirable. In fact, you should find the repetition more and more useful as you progress through the book.)

THE TECHNIQUE AND OTHER METHODS

People who have not had practical experience of the Technique often try to assess it by comparing it with something they know already, such as yoga, tai chi, biofeedback, and so on. There may well be points of contact between the Technique and these other disciplines, but what defines the Technique is what is unique to it, rather than what it shares with other systems.

If you practise yoga or another discipline and wish to compare it with the Alexander Technique, draw a list of its basic principles, and compare them with the principles of the Technique as discussed throughout this book. You will then see what they share and what is unique to each.

Ideally, you should acquaint yourself with the Alexander Technique without pre-conceived ideas. Go through the practical experiences offered by lessons in the Technique with an open mind, and let your intellectual understanding of the Technique and its principles flow naturally from these experiences.

CHAPTER 2
The Use of the Self

POSTURE

Take a few moments to think about posture. What does 'good posture' mean? Can you think of a few examples of people with good posture? Describe one such person in detail. Contrast, in your mind, 'good posture' and 'bad posture'. Can you pinpoint the differences between the two? How is good posture acquired? How is it lost? What are the effects of posture, good or bad, on health and well-being?

The way you answer the preceding questions reveals much about your understanding of how human beings move, react, and live. More usefully, it gives us some pointers on both how you live yourself and how you think you *should* live, for your conception of 'posture' entails a model of daily living.

For the sake of argument, imagine that you think that you have bad posture, and that you believe that classical dancers always have good posture. Now imagine that you think that your bad posture may be causing some health problems – backache, for example – and imagine too that you feel that your posture is bad because your back muscles are weak. If you start wishing to improve your posture, you may well be tempted to imitate the way a dancer stands or moves. You may even take dance classes or join a gym, with the express purpose of strengthening your postural muscles.

The above scenario illustrates many current attitudes about the body, as well as posture, tension, relaxation, strength, exercise, and health. Innocuous as they may seem, these attitudes determine a practical course of action – taking dance classes, for instance, or joining a gym. If one or more of these attitudes are mistaken, however, the course of action itself risks being mistaken and perhaps even harmful.

Whether you share these attitudes or not, it is useful to discuss them, for Alexander's views of the issues are in direct contrast to assumptions that are commonly perceived as being 'true'. By changing or discarding certain attitudes, you would logically change or discard your course of action. Therefore, this discussion has all-important practical consequences.

One dictionary definition of posture is 'the position or bearing of the body whether characteristic or assumed for a special purpose'. It is a simple definition that serves our purposes admirably. Other people may define posture more narrowly, as 'the position of the body'.

Two problems arise when we consider posture as a bodily position. The first is that this approach does not allow for the fact that there is no separation between the body and the mind, or between the 'physical' and the 'mental' (*see* Chapter 1). Posture, good or bad, is simply the outward manifestation of a series of convictions and beliefs. In truth, posture is synonymous with attitude. This is implicitly acknowledged by language: we speak of somebody's political posture, or use the word to describe the attitude of a musician at his instrument. It is useful to make this connection explicit, and always think of posture and attitude interchangeably. This will help you conceive of posture as an aspect of your whole being, not relating to your body alone. Such a conception may in turn lead you to seek 'good posture' in a more constructive manner than you would by simply thinking of bodily positions.

MOBILITY AND RESISTANCE

When you conceive of posture as a bodily position, you face a second problem – it assumes that there is an opposition between position and movement. You may think, for instance, that while standing you are in a position, and while walking you are moving. The risk then arises that you will seek good posture by holding yourself in a fixed position, changing it only long enough to assume a different (but equally fixed) position – from sitting to standing, for example. The American biologist George Coghill, a supporter of Alexander, wrote in one of Alexander's books that 'the distinction between mobility and immobility is relative, and no absolute distinction can be made between them'. He gave the example of deep sleep, a condition illustrative of immobility, and pointed out that, even then, 'the individual is mobilized in regard to its visceral, circular, and respiratory functions and the like'. Unless you are physically restrained, posture and movement are just two aspects of the same state of mobility. Coghill wrote that 'in posture the individual is as truly active as in movement … One phase passes over imperceptibly into the other'.[5]

The pianist and teacher Heinrich Neuhaus wrote that 'the best position of the hand on the keyboard is one which can be altered with the maximum of ease and speed.'[6] I believe that this applies usefully to all positions of the body, or to 'good posture', which is not a state of fixity, but one in which mobility is either latent or realized. This does not mean that you should move incessantly. Indeed, some people move too much, in harmful ways, and often without being aware of their movements – perhaps to counteract an uncomfortable rigidity. Latent mobility means simply that you should be able to move easily and elegantly at all times, if you wish to, or if the situation demands it. Latent mobility also means that you may be comfortable not moving at all, even for extended periods of time – for example, sitting listening to a lecture. Finally, latent mobility means that you may pass from rest to movement and to rest again with ease, slowly or quickly, consciously or by reflex, in innumerable ways according to need, desire, impulse, intuition, and imagination.

Mobility is not the be-all and end-all of good posture. Imagine an able basketball player in the midst of a competitive game. Even as he moves, he always retains the ability to resist other players' attempts to stop him, to unbalance him, or to push him out of the way. In effect, his mobility springs from a well of deep stability, and is in no way contradictory to it. Good posture, then, entails latent or realized mobility and latent or realized resistance.

Imagine that we are walking along together. Suddenly, you lean on me, putting your whole weight on my body, perhaps because you slipped and lost your balance momentarily. I am able to take your weight, not lose my own balance, and help you regain yours, however suddenly and heavily you have leant on me. This is because I use myself well, and I am permanently ready to resist a force that acts upon my body; that is, I have latent resistance. If you lean on me, this resistance –

fully operational at all times – becomes realized. I need it to push a door open, to carry a rucksack on my back or a heavy weight on my arms, to head a soccer ball into the net, and, indeed, for most activities of daily life, for work, rest, and play.

I do not need the presence of an outside force acting upon me to use my capacity to resist. Chapter 1 introduced the idea of the Primary Control – the orientation of the head in relation to the neck and back. For my spine to be as powerful and elastic as that of a seagull in flight, I direct my head forward and up, away from my back. At the same time I also direct my back backward and up, away from my head, thereby creating an opposition between the head (which goes forwards and up) and the back (which goes backwards and up). All parts of my body are in constant opposition to each other: the head to the back, the back to the arms, the elbows to the wrists, the wrists to the fingers, and so on. This opposition gives tonus to my body, lengthens and widens my back, and increases my strength, balance, and agility. Even as I sit quietly, not doing anything, I set antagonistic pulls throughout my body – in a sense, *I resist myself*.

As practised in the Alexander Technique, resistance, opposition, and antagonistic pulls are health-giving life forces, free from the negative connotations that these words may suggest in a different context. However, it is important to keep in mind that these pulls are not the result of something that you do, but rather of something that you stop doing. For more on this, *see* Chapter 3.

USE AND POSTURE

Alexander's concept of the 'use of the self' encompasses posture and goes beyond it at the same time. We know that language

shapes thought as much as thought shapes language; the way you think, speak, and act shows their mutual influence. Precisely because of the dangers of thinking of posture as represented by rigid bodily positions, it may be useful for you to think and speak not of good posture but of good use; and not of the way you use your body but of the way you use yourself.

It is possible for somebody to have bad posture (as 'posture' is generally understood), but to show good use as defined by Alexander. By virtue of a birth defect or an accident, a man's back may be bent and asymmetrical. Yet, if such a man directs his energies intelligently, he will be healthier than somebody who looks straight and symmetrical (and is therefore considered to have 'good posture'), but end-gains and over-reacts in a given situation. Many classical dancers appear to have good posture. Nevertheless, as you become better acquainted with the principles of the Alexander Technique, you will begin to notice that dancers do in fact use themselves quite badly, both on and off the stage. They also have to contend with serious health problems, during their careers and after retiring. If you are to abandon a rigid and narrow notion of posture, you will also need to give up seeing dancers as models of good posture. It goes without saying that there are marvellous dancers who use themselves exceptionally well; as previously mentioned, Fred Astaire was a paragon of elegance and good health into his old age.

It is possible to have good posture yet behave in an unintelligent manner. A serious Alexandrian would consider that such a person uses himself or herself badly. Here is a case in point.

Imagine a meeting, in which six or eight people are talking about politics. One of the participants sits quietly. He listens to everybody else carefully, thinks twice before saying anything, asks the meeting's chair for permission before he speaks, addresses the issue at hand without raising his voice or attacking other participants, makes his assumptions explicit, defines his terms precisely, and refers specific points to general principles. In sum, he behaves in a constructive and intelligent manner. Another participant fidgets throughout the meeting, talks to his neighbours, interrupts other speakers, raises unimportant points, speaks inarticulately, and makes personal attacks on people with whom he disagrees.

The first person may have a curved back and slumped shoulders (seen as 'bad posture'), while the second has square shoulders and a straight back ('good posture'), yet it is the first who is using himself well, and the second who is using himself badly. The first 'inhibits and directs' – two Alexandrian concepts discussed in Chapter 3 – while the second end-gains. It is worth making the point again, that thinking, speaking, and acting together constitute the way you use yourself, which goes well beyond posture, and all that 'posture' means.

INTELLIGENCE

The example above may lead to another conclusion about use, posture, and intelligence. Defining intelligence is very difficult. For a long time, intelligence was equated with academic ability, as measured by IQ tests. More recently, the concept of multiple intelligences, first advocated by Howard Gardner of Harvard University, has began to earn wide acceptance. By this measure of intelligence, Beethoven, Einstein, Freud, and Isadora Duncan, to name four outstanding people, would all be regarded as very intelligent. However, each would represent a particular type of intelligence: musical, academic, interrelational, and kinaes-

thetic. (According to Gardner, there are other types of intelligence as well as these.)

A broad and multi-layered definition of intelligence is both more true to intelligence itself and more useful for the practical purposes of change, growth, and the fulfilment of human potential. For the serious Alexandrian, intelligence in its multiple manifestations is a function of the way you use yourself, and a concrete phenomenon rather than an abstract concept. You are intelligent if you live intelligently; and you live intelligently if you use yourself well, like the first participant in the hypothetical meeting described above. Incidentally, such a person is more likely to examine himself and the world around him dispassionately, therefore accepting new ideas more openly. Even if he is an inept dancer or sportsman, he would still make a better Alexander pupil than a cocky athlete who lacks a measure of composure or detachment.

The way you use yourself affects your entire emotional state (*see* Chapter 5). Negative emotional states – bad moods, let us call them – are notorious for their keen effects on a person's intelligence. Do you do foolish things when you are in a bad mood? You may burn a piece of toast, drop a plate, cut your finger, forget your appointments, or say something you regret later. If you 'do' dumb things, it is because you have temporarily 'become' dumb. Logically enough, if under certain circumstances you can 'become' dumb and 'do' dumb things, under other circumstances you can 'become' intelligent and 'do' intelligent things. By using yourself well you will be, if not always in a good mood, then at least in an even one. Therefore, even if you do not become more intelligent after lessons in the Alexander Technique, at least you will start doing fewer foolish things.

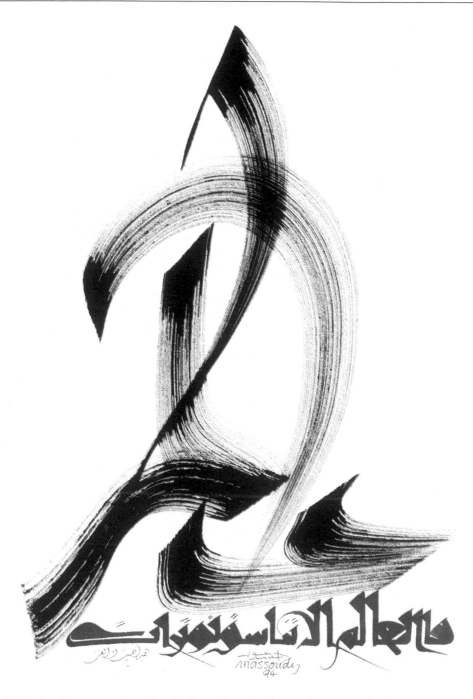

'The World is a Harmony of Tensions' – Heraclites of Ephesus. Drawing and calligraphy by Hassan Massoudy.

TENSION AND RELAXATION

The person who thinks about body positions almost inevitably thinks of tension and relaxation too. Just as received ideas about posture may harm you as you seek to improve your health, so would common conceptions of tension and relaxation.

'I am tense, I need to relax.' A simple statement of a simple observation, this little phrase – readily understood by all – contains a couple of assumptions that may stand in the way of your own health and well-being. The first assumption is that tension is inherently negative; in this case, 'to be tense' would always be wrong and undesirable. The second assumption is that, inversely, 'to be relaxed' would always be considered a positive thing. And a third assumption follows naturally: the remedy for tension is relaxation.

Imagine a horse being ridden by a man of medium build who weighs around 70kg (over 11 stones). Despite this heavy load on its back, the horse can run long distances at fast speeds, jumping over high fences and wide ditches, and up and down a mountain.

Imagine a violin. It has four strings, attached to pegs in a peg box up on the scroll of the instrument and to the tailpiece wrapped around the violin's base. These strings bear upon the bridge of the violin with enough force to strangle a man if applied to his throat. Besides the tension of the strings themselves, the violin also receives the pressure of the violinist's bow arm. Yet the violin thrives under this enormous tension, lasting unharmed for hundreds of years.

Picture a suspension bridge over a wide river. Every day, thousands of cars, trucks, and buses cross over it. At any one time, there may be several thousand tons bearing down upon this bridge. Yet it stands, strong and safe, year after year, without buckling or ever giving way.

The horse, the violin, and the bridge have several things in common. They are able to withstand enormous pressure. They are strong and durable. Although the rider, the violinist, and the engineer have different criteria, each would speak of the horse, the violin, and the bridge as being 'healthy': a healthy animal, a healthy instrument, and a healthy construction.

Have you ever run your hand down the vertebral column of a cat or a dog? When you apply pressure upon its spine, rather than yielding to the pressure, the cat will firm itself up, perhaps arching its back upwards, or perhaps just standing still and strong, purring contentedly even as you apply considerable force. The feeling of a spine that is firmed like this is not one of relaxation, but of proper tension – the right kind of tension, in the right places, in the right amount, for the right length of time. Indeed, what gives a cat its strength, agility, power, suppleness, and speed – its overall health – is this proper tension.

The horse loves its rider. Every day as it is taken out of the stable, the horse kicks its legs with joy in anticipation of being ridden – that is, of being made to bear great pressure on its back. If its rider were to stop riding it for a while, the horse would suffer as a result.

If you were to undo the tension of the violin strings and keep the instrument locked in a cupboard, untouched, for a few years, it would lose its capacity to vibrate to the touch of a bow. Musicians talk of their instruments as being 'happy' or 'unhappy'. My cello, for instance, 'loves' humidity, and is 'unhappy' in dry, heated rooms in winter. A string instrument, like a cat or a horse, is happy when it is under tension, and unhappy otherwise. Like a cat and a horse, like a magnificent Stradivarius or a gleaming Steinway, like a great suspension bridge, you will be happy and healthy not when you are relaxed, but when you have within you the *right tension*. That tension will make you vibrate and kick your legs in the air with joy. Once you have the right tension within you, you will be happier and healthier, and this will enable you to respond to all sorts of stimulations that engage and heighten your inner tension.

As you read these arguments in favour of tension, you may be inclined to counter that you think of cats – as well as dogs and horses, and other animals – as being perfectly relaxed. You might imagine that, if we humans should draw inspiration from them, it is their marvellous capacity for relaxation that we ought to imitate.

Because a cat has the support and vitality of a strong spine, its neck, shoulders, and limbs need a minimum amount of effort to do the work they are required to do. If we could artificially weaken the spine of a cat, it would have to use its neck, shoulders, and limbs more actively and forcefully than it does naturally. In such a state, the cat would give a fair imitation of a badly co-ordinated human being at work – awkward, inefficient, and inelegant. Relaxation, in an animal or in a human being, is a side-effect of proper tension. Conversely, too much tension is a side-effect of the absence of *proper* tension. A seemingly perfectly relaxed cat is in fact in a state of perfectly balanced tension.

Picture a recent occasion when you felt that you were too tense, perhaps an afternoon at the office when the workload was too heavy and you felt 'under stress', a long day's shopping in a crowded department store, typing at a computer, driving or riding a car, or a Sunday evening after a game of competitive soccer with friends. Perhaps, even as you read this book (maybe you are sitting in a café), you feel uncomfortable and distracted by a nagging pull in the back of your neck.

In any of these situations, if you think that too much tension is the cause of your discomfort, you are likely to pursue its contrary – relaxation – as an antidote. Yet, as you work, shop, play, ride, and read, you misuse and overuse certain parts of your body (your neck and shoulders, for example) to compensate for misusing and *under-using* other parts (the back and legs, for example). It is the absence of the right kind of tension in the right places for the right length of time that causes too much tension of the wrong kind in the wrong places for the wrong length of time, as illustrated by the weakened cat in our imaginary experiment. If, as you try to relax wrong tensions in the neck and shoulders, you further relax your spine, you are likely to create even greater wrong tensions. Badly conceived and directed, relaxation is then a problem, not a solution.

Let us recapitulate briefly. The way you use yourself encompasses posture and goes beyond it. Your posture is inseparable from your attitude; indeed, the two are synonymous. It is possible to use yourself well while giving the impression to others that you have bad posture. Inversely, it is possible to appear to have good posture and yet use yourself badly. A good position is that which you can alter with the greatest speed and ease. If you use yourself well, you pass from posture to movement and back to posture again easily, quickly, and imperceptibly. You have latent resistance and latent mobility at all times, and you activate each as needed, in turn and together. 'Too much tension' is better expressed as 'too much wrong tension', that is, wrong in kind, amount, place, and time. The cause of wrong tension is the absence of right tension, and true relaxation is a side-effect of the latter. Finally, to be intelligent means to live intelligently, and to live intelligently means using yourself well.

CHAPTER 3
Inhibition and Direction

REACTING TO A STIMULUS

I am giving my pupil Estelle an Alexander lesson. I ask her to watch me as I take three juggling balls in my hands and juggle them for ten or fifteen seconds. Without any further instructions, I hand the balls to Estelle and ask her to juggle.

'I can't do it,' she replies at once. 'I haven't got a knack for this sort of thing.' It is obvious from her demeanour and her tone of voice that she is terrified of juggling, or, more precisely, of the *idea* of trying to juggle. Yet Estelle is a professional singer who can perform complex musical pieces in front of an audience. In her daily life she is perfectly able to drive a car in hectic traffic and talk with a passenger at the same time. She is comfortable riding a bicycle in the countryside, sometimes carrying her shopping or one of her children with her. She tends a large garden where her co-ordination is challenged in many different ways, and she often accomplishes admirable botanical feats balancing herself in acrobatic positions for a long while. In short, her current psychomotor abilities are quite impressive. Why, then, is she so sure that she will not be able to perform the simple gestures that juggling requires, and why does she express her certainty with such anxiety?

Most people judge themselves all the time, and, perhaps without being aware of it, think also that they are being judged by others all the time. Think about this for a moment: if most people are constantly worrying about being judged by others, they will not be spending very much time judging others. Thinking that others are judging you, and fearing their judgements, are two symptoms of an unwarranted and unhealthy self-centredness. Estelle's unconscious fear of being judged by me while she tries to juggle is not justified.

In fact, I do not judge Estelle; rather, I observe her. It is true that, as I observe her juggling, I could easily arrive at certain conclusions about some other of her behaviours, perhaps even about her whole being. After all, juggling stands as a sort of metaphor for life; that is the reason why juggling is so useful in an Alexander lesson. Even then, however, Estelle's fear of juggling and of being judged would not be justified. I know her well, I have often expressed my appreciation of her many attributes, and I always speak to her with respect and affection. She knows that I am 'for' her, not 'against' her. Still, despite all the rational arguments that could be presented in this situation, Estelle is afraid of juggling because she is afraid of being judged.

Another reason why Estelle is so anxious is her fear of failure. Indeed, she is absolutely convinced that she *will* fail. However, in this instance, she is convinced of a fact that has not come into existence, for she declares her inability to juggle before throwing a single ball up in the air. In a sense, it might be possible to say that she 'wants' to fail.

To explain this point, I must make a detour.

I was an extremely awkward and sedentary child, and only learned to ride a bicycle as a young adult, at the time when I was starting to take lessons in the Alexander Technique. After receiving some instruction from my girl-friend, I went to practise, wobbling on the bike around a public square. Once, I tried to cross the square instead of going around it. There was a lamp post right in the middle; I saw it from a distance and started to worry about riding into it, despite all the empty space around it. I found myself saying, in my mind, 'I'm going to hit it! I'm going to hit it!' This was an expression of my fear of hitting it, but my words indicate not only that I wanted to hit the post, but also that I was determined to do so – as I inevitably did.

Estelle is anxious for a third reason: she is afraid of the unknown. She has never juggled in her life, and naturally knows nothing about the mechanics of juggling. A number of other situations might trigger in her a similar disqui-et, such as finding herself in a group of people she has not met before, suffering from some illness without knowing its diagnosis or prog-nosis, or moving house. Faced with juggling for the first time, Estelle is not so much afraid of juggling itself as of something she has never encountered before. Alexander liked to say that, at the very heart of his technique, there was the journey that the pupil must make from the known into the unknown, the known being wrong and the unknown right.

Estelle's fear of juggling, of being judged, of failing, and of facing the unknown all cause her to tense up in such a way that she makes it hard for herself to learn how to juggle. Jug-gling becomes truly difficult, thereby justify-ing her fear of it in some way. My job as an Alexander teacher is not so much to show her how to juggle, but to help her lose her fear of the unknown. Alexander neatly summed up the nature of a lesson: 'You are not here to do exercises, or to learn to do something right,

but to get able to meet a stimulus that always puts you wrong and to learn to deal with it.'[7] When I ask Estelle to juggle, I am putting her somehow 'in the wrong', but only so that I can start helping her learn to deal with it.

Here we come to an important reason why Estelle is so afraid. Because of her habit of end-gaining, she has misunderstood the pur-pose of the exercise. The basics of juggling are very simple. The number of things that you can do with a juggling ball is limited: you can throw it up in the air, catch it with either hand, throw it sideways from one hand direct-ly into the other, hold it in your hand – and not much else. It is true that, once you start performing these motions with three balls in alternation, in combination, and in sequence, the possibilities are vast, yet one fact remains. This is that the basic motions are all extreme-ly simple. When you combine these motions in twos, threes, and more, the resulting activ-ity is complex rather than complicated. At its core it retains the simplicity of the first, easy straightforward throw. If you can pass a ball from one hand to the other, you can juggle. Yet, simple as juggling itself may be, the main purpose of the exercise is not for you to learn how to juggle. Before considering the real reason why I have asked Estelle to juggle, let us first look at how Estelle goes about it.

END-GAINING AND MISUSE

I show Estelle the eight or ten steps that would take her from throwing a single ball up in the air to juggling three balls at the same time and continuously. The first step is to throw a ball up in the air, without even trying to catch it. The second step is to throw a ball up in the air, and catch it with your other hand. The third step is to throw a ball up in the air from your left hand; as it goes up and reaches the highest point of its flight, throw a ball up in the air from your right hand, without trying to catch either ball. The fourth step is the same as the previous one, but now try to catch, with one hand, the second ball you threw from your other hand. The steps continue in this fashion, becoming ever more complex until you actually find yourself juggling.

When Estelle attempts the first, very simple, step, she misuses her whole self as she throws the ball up in the air. She pulls her head back and down into her neck, lifts her shoulders, pushes her pelvis forward, and stops breathing. Needless to say, she is not aware of any of these misuses. Her sole concern is to 'do the right thing' and throw the ball up in the air. She thinks only of the end, and neglects the means whereby she could attain that end. As she goes on to the following steps, her misuse becomes ever worse. Remember the description of the first few steps of juggling: you throw one or two balls in the air without actually trying to catch them. Estelle finds this extremely hard to do; she is so intent on catching the balls that she often fails to throw them up in the air to begin with!

Here, Estelle reveals how she end-gains and misunderstands the nature of the exercise. Indeed, she misunderstands the nature of juggling itself. For Estelle – as for most pupils who try to juggle for the first time – juggling means *catching* balls. She is so eager to do this that she ends up not throwing the balls at all, but she cannot catch something that she has not thrown. The definition that Estelle applies to juggling ('catching balls') prevents her from juggling (in other words, throwing and possibly catching balls).

More importantly, however, Estelle misunderstands the nature of the situation in which she finds herself. My asking her to juggle was a pretext, a ruse and a trap. The true purpose of the exercise is more subtle than it appears. First, I would like Estelle to become aware of her reactions; second, to become aware of her

end-gaining; third, to become aware of her misuses; fourth, to stop her end-gaining; fifth, to stop her misuse, which is a consequence of her end-gaining; and sixth, to juggle. However, even if she is unable to juggle at the end of the lesson, she may still have accomplished what I hoped for her; if she becomes better aware of her own reactions, the first purpose of the exercise will have been achieved.

Some pupils, like Estelle, will spend long sessions trying to juggle, during which time they pay no attention whatsoever to their use. Such people have fallen into the trap. As long as Estelle's main concern is to juggle three balls (the presumed end of the exercise), she will neglect the double means whereby the end may be achieved. The means include, on the one hand, the intermediate steps of throwing one or two balls without trying to catch them, and, on the other hand, Estelle's awareness of the way she uses herself. Her use comprises the co-ordination of her whole body from head to toe, and also her attitudes and beliefs, her reactions, and her habits of thought and action.

As she attempts to juggle, Estelle end-gains to an extraordinary degree, and, because she end-gains, she misuses herself badly. I ask her simply to drop the balls; she always tries to catch them, twisting her body in the process. I ask her not to pick up the balls that fall on the floor, and beg her to let me pick them up for her instead. Again and again, she drops a ball and immediately reaches down for it. Then I ask her to stop for a brief moment after dropping a ball, and consider the co-ordination of her gestures before picking it up. Even though the instructions are freshly repeated every minute, Estelle reacts too soon and too fast, and 'forgets' to co-ordinate herself every time she drops a ball and reaches down for it. When she drops a ball, she exclaims, angry with herself, 'No!' I point out to her that her expression of dissatisfaction is disproportionate to the situation; after all, this is only a game. In addition, Estelle's expression of dissatisfaction – a brusque and emphatic gesture of her head, which shortens her neck and spine – contributes to her misuse and makes it more likely that she miss subsequent catches. (In this matter, she has two choices: not to express her frustration, or not to become frustrated. One of these choices is clearly superior to the other.)

Estelle's eagerness to throw and catch the balls 'in the right way' creates such tensions that she throws the balls awkwardly and drops them every time. Because she end-gains, she misuses herself in such a manner that she becomes unable to attain her desired goal. Therefore, for her to be able to catch the balls, she must stop being so eager to catch them; for her to be able to juggle, she must give up the wish to juggle.

PAYING ATTENTION TO THE MEANS

I ask Estelle to slow down her actions and to repeat a simple gesture once, twice, three times – for instance, throwing a single ball from one hand to the other. At times, I hold her hands and prevent her from juggling, and ask her simply to listen to me as I explain something, or watch me as I demonstrate a technique. I reassure her again and again that she has the right to drop one or more balls without worrying and, above all, without reproaching herself. Estelle is so hypnotized by her wish to do the right thing that she becomes incapable of talking to me, looking at me, or listening to me when I address her. I ask her to keep eye contact with me, to walk around the room, or to move her head as she speaks – anything to break her hypnotic state and to help her recover her reason.

From time to time, I stop the exercise altogether, and ask Estelle to clear her mind of her anxieties and preconceived ideas about the difficulty of the task and her inability to perform it. To mitigate her frustration with herself, I ask her to alternate her efforts at juggling with other activities that she has mastered, so that she can remind herself of how accomplished she really is. I ask her to hear her own manner of speaking about herself – 'I can't do it,' 'Damn it!,' 'NO!' – and I encourage her to speak to herself and about herself with all the tenderness that she deserves. We talk, joke, and laugh. I persuade her that I do not expect her to juggle or to 'do well'; instead, all I ask is that she observe herself in all her actions.

I ask her to touch me as I juggle, and feel the stability and strength of my body. I give her suggestions on how to use her arms and hands. I use my hands to touch Estelle as she juggles, and direct her attention to various parts of her body – her head, her neck, her back, her shoulders, her pelvis. I use words as well as my hands, and help Estelle associate a set of words, a psycho-physical experience, and the feedback she receives from it. Later, Estelle will use these words as reminders of the physical experiences. Little by little we train her muscular memory, so that one day she will be able to move freely by using the verbal instructions we cultivated as she juggled:

'Let your neck be free.'
'Direct your head forward and up.'
'Let your back lengthen and widen.'
'Stay in your back.'
'Point up along the spine.'
'Drop your shoulders and point them out, away from each other.'
'Don't sway your pelvis.'
'Don't freeze your eyes, and remember to blink regularly.'
'Don't forget to breathe.' 'Don't force your breathing.'
'Stay out of the way.'

When Estelle tries too hard to interpret my directions muscularly, she misuses herself even more. I say to her, 'Let your neck be free.' Immediately she starts to move her head in an attempt to free her neck, but the more she moves her head, the stiffer her neck becomes. I suggest to her not *to do* these directions, but *to let them be* instead. I explain that most of these directions are not orders for her to do something ('lift an arm', for instance, or 'grab a ball'), but orders for her to stop doing something ('release your shoulders') or for her to prevent herself from doing something ('don't tighten your shoulders').

As her will turns away from juggling and towards her own use, Estelle goes through a complete transformation. She loses her anxiety and begins to smile and laugh, even as she drops a ball. Her discourse changes. She stops saying, 'I can't do this,' or 'This is impossible.' She also stops chiding herself and letting out exclamations of frustration such as 'NO!' or 'Damn!' Instead, she finds herself saying, 'Hey, this is fun!'

She stops making wild grabs for balls that fall too far for her to catch them. She stops twisting her body into awkward positions, throwing her head back and down, lifting her shoulders, and swaying her pelvis. Instead, she stands still, stable but not rigid, and uses her arms lightly and elegantly. Watching her, one has the impression that she is doing something simple, easy, and enjoyable.

To her own surprise, she finds herself catching balls seemingly without the participation of her conscious will; the balls fall into her hands and the juggling does itself, so to speak. She forgets the very idea of doing well, of success and failure. Instead of judging herself or fearing others' judgements, she observes herself in action, dispassionately, yet full of curiosity and good humour. She acts without concerning herself with the results of her actions.

If we compare Estelle as she was earlier on in her Alexander lesson and as she is now, we see that she has become a different person altogether. It is not simply that she uses her body in a more relaxed manner. Her gestures are now animated by entirely different thoughts and desires. Earlier, her reactions to the situation with which I had presented her – an invitation to juggle – were wholly unjustified and inappropriate. What should have been a simple exercise in psychomotor skills had been in effect a threatening and painful challenge to her whole person. As Estelle lets go of her first, automatic, habitual impulses (of which she was not aware), her reactions become healthy, reasonable, well-thought-out, constructive, and practical.

INHIBITION AND DIRECTION

This is a good point at which to recapitulate and define the basic principles of the Alexander Technique.

- We do not use or misuse our bodies; we use or misuse ourselves. On the one hand, our thoughts, assumptions, suppositions and beliefs all play a rôle in our use and misuse. Estelle's use includes matters of will, control, judgement, anger and frustration. On the other hand, our entire body, from head to toe, is present in everything that we do, whether we do it well or badly. As Estelle juggles, she misuses her head, neck, back, shoulders, arms, torso, legs and feet, as well as her eyes, her breathing mechanisms, and much else besides. Inversely, when she stops end-gaining and invests herself fully in the means whereby she may achieve her ends, she uses her whole self well.
- We misuse ourselves in most of what we do. We do so habitually, and without being

aware of it. In previous chapters we discussed proprioception, misuse, and habit, and we can now include 'will' in this equation. Estelle is not aware of her behaviours, hypnotized as she is by her 'will to do well'. The more she misuses herself, the less aware she becomes of her misuses, and the more unaware she is of her misuse, the worse the misuse becomes.

- We misuse ourselves for many different reasons. Yet the most important reason for our misuse – important because of its practical consequences and because we can do something about it – is our habit of end-gaining. When she juggles, Estelle misuses herself because she goes directly and intensely for a desired end (catching balls) rather than paying attention to the means necessary for her to accomplish what she has set out to do.

- To stop misusing herself, Estelle has no choice but to stop end-gaining. Alexander called this process – of consciously giving up end-gaining habits and reactions – 'inhibition'.

- Consciously and unconsciously, we give ourselves orders, or 'directions', all the time. When Estelle says 'I can't,' or 'NO!', she is giving herself directions to act in a certain way, and her directions result in a psycho-physical state. We also give ourselves directions without words.

- Directions are messages from the brain to the muscles, via the nerves. Just as we give ourselves directions when misusing ourselves, we can also use them to inhibit end-gaining habits and reactions, and to stop misusing ourselves. Carefully chosen and interpreted, these directions – verbal or not – serve the purpose of stopping us from doing too much too soon, or simply from doing it badly.

- The most useful directions inhibit action, rather than excite it; they are orders to *stop* doing. Since the orientation of the head, neck, and back determines the co-ordination of the whole body, the most important directions are those that stop you from misusing your Primary Control. We can call these 'primary directions'. It does not matter what situation you find yourself in – learning to juggle, handling stage fright, dealing with conflict; your inhibiting starts with your primary directions.

- When we inhibit end-gaining habits and reactions, we get the impression that we are *doing nothing*, and that things *do themselves*. When Estelle juggles without end-gaining, she has the feeling that balls fall into her hands as if in the absence of her conscious will. In fact, Estelle is doing quite a lot of things when she inhibits, but these are of a different nature from her usual muscular exertions. Inhibiting does not entail becoming passive or complacent. Rather, to inhibit is not to do anything unnecessary, excessive, unreasonable, or harmful. This leaves us free to do everything that is necessary, well-measured, reasonable, and healthy.

- Juggling in Estelle's lesson stands as a metaphor for every human activity. Her behaviours as she juggles are typical of her style of daily living and interpersonal relationships; they are 'normal' for her. This is discussed further in Chapter 4, where 'normal' behaviours are contrasted with 'natural' ones.

- In every situation we face, we can either use ourselves well or misuse ourselves; we can be unreasonable and unhealthy, or reasonable and healthy. In short, we can end-gain and mis-direct ourselves, or we can inhibit and direct ourselves adequately. Inhibition and direction, two inseparable facets of the same human capability, are the key to the Alexander Technique. Indeed, without them it is impossible for us to pass from using ourselves badly to using ourselves well. When we inhibit, we lose the fear of being judged, the fear of failing, and the fear of the unknown. To pass from the known to the unknown is the most important, difficult, and wonderful journey in our life.

DIRECTIONS AND WORDS

It is possible to give directions without using words, and to use words without sending directions. People who are naturally well co-ordinated – for example, small children – give themselves directions without using words, and perhaps without knowing that they are, indeed, directing their use. All the same, well-chosen and constructively applied words can be an excellent tool for learning how to direct your use.

Alexander used the following phrasing for the primary directions: 'Let your neck be free, to let your head go forward and up, to let the back lengthen and widen, all together, one after the other.'

Note that the success of the entire formulation hinges on the word 'let'. You cannot *make* your neck be free – that would be a contradiction in terms. Note too that the directions are so interconnected as to create a working unity; if you neglect one of the directions, the whole suffers. Directions have hierarchy and order: freeing the neck precedes letting the head go forward and up. Yet it is important to give your directions 'all together, one after the other', and not in isolation from each other. To direct is to co-ordinate yourself, and as the word itself implies, co-ordination entails many parts working together harmoniously.

The primary directions are inhibitory – orders to stop doing or not to do – and need not result in muscular activity. Think of them as double negatives, or the contrary of something undesirable. A free neck is one that is not tightened; to let the head go forward and up is to prevent it from bearing back and down on the neck; to lengthen and widen the back is to prevent it from shortening and narrowing. However, if you try to lengthen and widen your back wilfully, you are likely to stiffen your neck in the process. What makes a neck stiff is too much activity; the contrary of too much activity is not more activity, but its cessation. To repeat, 'to let' is the key that unlocks the chain.

When something upsets your inner balance – for example, if you are startled by a car backfiring – a single, sudden thought makes you misuse your whole self. Ideally, a single thought of a different kind should also trigger all the directions that establish the best use of your whole self. However, until you can summon such a thought, you will need to pay attention to each direction in turn. In time, you will discover the words (or thoughts, or images) that awaken your good use. My favourite trigger is simple: 'Think up'.

CHAPTER 4
The Lesson

THE ESSENCE OF A LESSON

There is no standard way of teaching the Alexander Technique. As in all other human activity, it is difficult, if not impossible, to separate the principles advocated by a professional from his personality, temperament, background, and much else besides. In other words, any set of principles can only be judged by the individual way in which they are practised. It could be argued that there has only ever been one Alexander teacher: F.M. Alexander himself. He trained many teachers, all of whom had his or her own understanding of the work. These teachers in turn have trained others, who again have brought their individual characteristics to the Technique. In sum, each teacher works in a manner unique to him or her, and the same teacher may also have a different approach for different pupils.

In this chapter I describe what I consider the logic underlying the work of an Alexander teacher during lessons. If you find a teacher whose methods do not correspond with my description, you will have to judge his or her merits and demerits for yourself, using my observations as well as your own critical sense. (At any rate, I expect you to use your discernment to consider the merits and demerits of everything I tell you!)

What defines the spirit of an Alexander lesson (as opposed to its form) is that it is indeed a *lesson*, and not a therapy or counselling or healing session. A learning process should always take place in an Alexander lesson, regardless of the reason – a breathing disorder, arthritis, or depression, for example – why the pupil has sought out a teacher. The aim of the Alexander teacher is not to treat or cure a patient, but to teach a pupil how to inhibit end-gaining habits and reactions, and how to direct the whole self, with particular emphasis on the Primary Control – the orientation of the head relative to the neck, and of both to the back.

The Technique has far-reaching therapeutic effects on both 'physical' and 'mental' illnesses, but these effects occur indirectly, as a result of the pupil's ability to prevent his or her habitual misuses. In attempting to affect an illness directly, both teacher and pupil may well end-gain and neglect the very processes which allow an illness to change and disappear.

In an Alexander lesson, you do not learn how to do the right thing; rather, you learn how to stop doing the wrong thing. Alexander used to say that, if you stop the wrong thing, the right thing will do itself. If your illness or discomfort is caused by something that you are doing, you cannot be 'cured' of it by any means other than stopping doing the thing that causes it. At all moments, teacher and pupil both must carry on with this learning process, which creates the conditions in which healing and cure happen by themselves.

THE 'NORMAL' AND THE 'NATURAL'

Lessons cover the two major aspects of activity and rest. Lessons may start with either, and may include either, or both. When a teacher chooses an activity in a lesson, the purpose is not so much to master the activity itself but to use it as a means to a greater end. Each activity becomes a laboratory where matters of awareness, reaction, use, and attitude may be examined; *see* the previous chapter, where juggling is used as an example.

In an Alexander lesson, the teacher presents the pupil with a stimulus, usually of a psychomotor nature; the pupil may be asked to sit, stand, lean forward or backward, turn his or her head, say a vowel or a word, walk, juggle, and so on. Each stimulus provokes many possible reactions in a pupil, but most reactions can be seen as either 'normal' or 'natural'.

Here, we need to define the above terms. (Too often, participants in a conversation use certain words or terms without considering that others may believe the same words to mean something different, or possibly even to have the opposite meaning.) 'Normal' may mean two distinct things:

1. according to an average; or
2. according to a model.

'Natural' may mean at least three different things:

1. habitual and unpremeditated;
2. removed from civilization or untouched by it; or
3. according to the laws of nature, intrinsically right.

For the purposes of the current discussion, let us define 'normal' reactions as according to an average – that is, based upon most people's reactions most of the time – and 'natural' as according to the laws of nature – based upon how most people's reactions *should ideally be* in the right conditions.

If you are presented with a stimulus, you can react normally (as you always have, and as most people would), or naturally (in the manner that best suits the situation). Let us imagine that I ask you to juggle. If you are like most people, you will become anxious and flustered, complicate a simple situation, end-gain, misuse your whole self, and fail miserably. This is normal, but in no way natural. My job as an Alexander teacher is to help you stop reacting normally, so that you may start reacting naturally to any situation with which you may be presented. If you react naturally, you will be able to juggle easily and with pleasure, and enjoy the learning process even if you fail to juggle.

In juggling, the distinction between normal and natural is very evident for most pupils to see. What they do not realize is that the same distinction exists for every single situation, reaction, thought, and gesture, including the simplest acts of daily life. Indeed, it is altogether unnecessary to introduce complex motor skills in a lesson for a pupil to pass from normal to natural or to learn the principles of the Technique; the whole learning experience can happen through the simple action of sitting and standing. However, keep in mind that the purpose of the lesson is not to teach you the right way of sitting and standing, but to help you pass from normal to natural, from the known to the unknown, from wrong to right, in *everything* you do, without exception.

As well as normal and natural reactions, there are also 'abnormal' reactions. Try the following experiment. Pull your head back and down in an exaggerated manner, so that you shorten your neck grievously. This is an 'abnormal' position that corresponds neither to an average nor to a model. While keeping your head in this position, say a few words. Undoubtedly you will be struck by how strange your voice sounds. Now, bring your head back to a normal position, and say the same words you said before. The use of your voice is clearly improved once you pass from the abnormal to the normal. You may now suppose that there must be a natural orientation of the head, superior to the normal one, in which the use of your voice would be yet healthier and freer.

It is relatively easy to pass from the abnormal to the normal. Passing from the normal to the natural is more difficult, both because of faulty sensory awareness, and because such a passage occurs not because of something that you do, but because of something that you stop doing.

The existence of abnormal reactions does not change the essence of an Alexander lesson, which remains the subtle and delicate passage from the normal to the natural. In any case, if you learn how to pass from the normal to the natural, you will know everything you need in order to pass easily from the abnormal to the normal.

STIMULUS AND REACTION

Every day, all day long, you react constantly to all sorts of stimuli: sensorial, intellectual, emotional. You react to other people, to situations, to wishes, to fears. You do so consciously or subconsciously, sometimes in a healthy manner, sometimes unhealthily. All that matters, though, is that you react nonstop, and always with your whole being.

In effect, the way you use yourself is actually the way you react to each and every

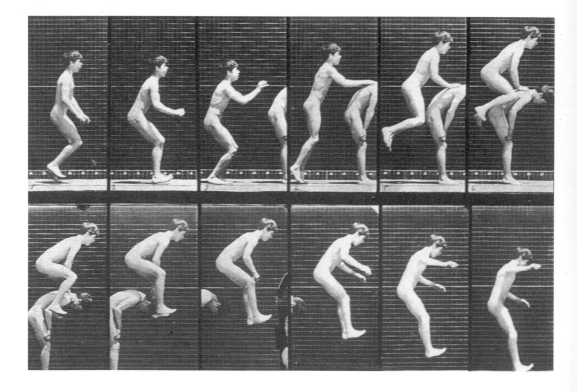

situation. The Alexander teacher bases his or her entire pedagogical work upon this simple observation. During a lesson, the teacher uses all sorts of means to make you react, thereby offering you the possibility of learning how to inhibit and direct. Although Alexander developed a number of traditional procedures, this does not mean that every teacher must work according to a set of formulas. It is possible to learn the principles of the Technique without ever making use of the traditional procedures, although they are particularly well suited to the purpose. (For a discussion of Alexander's procedures, *see* the end of this chapter.)

The rationale of a lesson is rather simple. As already noted, in every situation you react with your entire being; your reactions may be normal or natural. When you react normally, you react the way everybody else does, according to your habits, with little consciousness of your actions or control over them, with too much effort, in a hurry or hesitantly, in a manner that is inelegant, inefficient, and costly to your well-being. (Needless to say, because of faulty sensory perception, you may well be unaware of any of the characteristics of your normal reactions.) When you react naturally, you react according to the laws of nature, in an ideal manner, with a degree of awareness and control, aided at the same time by reasoning and intuition, in a manner that is adequate to the situation, using yourself with elegance and power.

The work of the teacher, then, is to make you react to various stimuli, and help you to pass in all your reactions from normal to natural. This all-important point may be illustrated by an exercise that I often use in my teaching practice.

We are both standing up. I place myself in front of you, put my hands on your shoulders, and make you lean forward, towards me. Your reaction to my gesture is multi-layered, and reveals much to me about your use – your 'character' and 'individuality', in Alexander's

words. You react to the situation itself, to my words, to my way of looking at you, to my hands on your shoulders, and, most importantly, to the movement of your body towards me. When I lean you forward, I make you lose your balance. More precisely, I put you in a position in which you think (or feel) that you are unbalanced; in fact, since I am holding you myself, you are perfectly balanced. I use my back and my legs – indeed, my whole body – in such a way that it is perfectly easy for me to hold you without effort, free from the risk of hurting myself or of letting you drop.

However, a feeling of imbalance, a fear of falling, a fear of not mastering the situation, and a lack of trust in me as I hold you will all lead you to misuse your whole self. You will pull your head backward, raise your shoulders, hollow your back, lock your knees, lift your heels off the ground, and hold your breath. This reaction of fear and misuse is absolutely normal: it mirrors other reactions of yours in different situations, and it mirrors the reactions of the vast majority of people who find themselves in this particular situation. In such a context, your reaction corresponds to an average, to a 'norm', but it is in no way natural. By definition, all that is natural is ideal. Your fear of falling and the contraction of your body caused by this fear cannot be ideal. They are not even justified, since I hold you surely and firmly, and I will not let you fall.

I now start to reassure you verbally. I do the exercise and its many variants several times. I explain and demonstrate. I bring your attention to the different ways you misuse your body. I help you inhibit and direct, and little by little you start changing your reaction to my stimulus. You redirect your head, release your shoulders, lengthen and widen your back, bring your heels down, start breathing freely, and become light and strong. You have finally accepted that you have nothing to fear, and your entire reaction becomes free from anxiety and contraction. You now react according to the requirements of the situation; you react naturally, not normally.

When you first do the exercise, you are most likely to believe that your first reaction, which we have called 'normal', is the only possible reaction given the situation in which you find yourself. The fear of falling is quite real; if you did fall, you would risk injuring yourself. As I take you off balance you contract yourself instinctively, to protect yourself from a dangerous fall. Your reaction then seems to you both necessary and inevitable, and you are tempted to say that the situation *causes* your reaction.

However, we have already determined that the situation is not at all unsafe, as I am holding you quite firmly. Your fear of falling is therefore unjustified, as is your manner of misusing your whole body. Let us go further down this line of reasoning. Every child falls regularly, usually without the least injury; so do dancers, clowns, martial artists, and athletes, as well as animals, both wild and domesticated. If you take a kitten in your hands and throw it up in the air, it will re-orientate itself as it falls, find its balance in mid-air, and land lightly on its paws.

In the above situation, you would risk nothing even if I did let you fall. Like the kitten, you can re-orient yourself and take a couple of steps forward, thereby regaining your balance; like the clown and the martial artist, you can take a fall with grace, and not hurt yourself. (Note that, in the case of a child or an animal, the ability to fall lightly is inborn; in the case of a dancer or an athlete, the ability is consciously developed. If you have lost your inborn ability – which you certainly had as a child – all you have to do is regain it with the help of your adult intelligence.)

You see now that your first reaction to my destabilizing gesture was doubly unjustified, both because you are perfectly balanced in my hands, and because falling can and should be a source of pleasure, not pain.

One winter day, coming out of the Van Gogh Museum in Amsterdam, I slipped on the icy sidewalk and fell on my backside. The fall took me by surprise, and seemed to last not more than a second. I did not have the time to choose my reaction, and yet I reacted in a wholly natural manner. In effect, I did not have the feeling of falling, but rather of flying, or of falling upwards. The experience was pleasant and amusing, and the recollection of this magical moment made me smile all day long. Needless to say, I did not hurt myself at all as I fell.

When I put you in a situation that seems to unbalance you, I help you work through several aspects of your being. First, we seek to eliminate an entirely unjustifiable fear – the fear of falling when, in truth, you are perfectly balanced. Second, we seek to develop the means required for you to react differently to a possibly, but not necessarily, justified fear – the fear of falling awkwardly and hurting yourself. As your co-ordination improves, you learn to fall upwards, instinctively like a kitten or a child, or intuitively like a dancer or a clown. (You may wish to reflect for a moment upon the difference between instinct and intuition.) At any rate, when you lose the fear of falling, or, more precisely, the fear of injuring yourself, you are more likely to have fewer accidents; if you have an accident, you are more likely to have fewer injuries: and, if you suffer an injury, you are more likely to recover more quickly from it.

The most useful lesson that you will learn from the experience of losing your balance in the hands of an Alexander teacher is that, in every situation, you have a range of possible reactions. You will then stop believing (and claiming) that a situation, a stimulus, or a person *causes* you to react in an inevitable manner. This should eventually lead to you mastering your reactions, and not being a slave to them.

THE LOGIC OF A LESSON

The choice of activities used in an Alexander lesson is only limited by the physical setting of the lesson and the imagination of the teacher. Teachers have used creeping and crawling, horse-riding, calligraphy, typewriting, speaking, singing, martial arts, rôle-playing, and much more. What matters is not the activity itself, but the way it is presented and handled by the teacher. A few points are in order.

Most of the time, there is a gap between what you are doing and what you think you are doing. This is the phenomenon of faulty sensory awareness. By touching you with my hands in certain specific ways, which is discussed below, I may be able to help you narrow and eventually eliminate this gap. This, inevitably, becomes difficult in a large group. The ideal way of teaching and learning the Technique is individually, and through activities that can be easily monitored and altered by the teacher's hands.

The more you have invested, personally and professionally, in a particular area of your life, the harder your habits in that area may be to change. If you are a pianist, for example, you will have spent long years cultivating your habits of playing; these habits will have muscular, aural, psychological and aesthetic components. Since you derive your identity as a person and as a professional from the way you play the piano, it may be easier for you to start learning the principles of the Technique away from your instrument. Ideally, lessons in the Technique should progress from the general to the particular, and in an increasing order of complexity. On the first count, the examination of everyday activities should precede any scrutiny of your professional habits and the learning of new skills. On the second count, sitting and standing should precede juggling. It is possible for a resourceful and conscientious pupil to apply the principles of the Technique to his or her every activity from the first lesson onwards, but the difficulties of doing this should not be underestimated.

The changes from normal to natural in your reactions happen through the twin processes of inhibition and direction. The more opportunities an activity presents for inhibition, the more useful this activity is in learning the Alexander Technique. Juggling offers many such opportunities (*see* Chapter 3). However, the stimulation of life is never-ending, and, therefore, the possibilities for inhibiting are also never-ending. The teacher may present to you a number of stimuli in succession: sit, stand, lean forward, turn your head, lift an arm, say a word. Each demands inhibition and direction. Soon you will realize that life itself invites you to inhibit and direct at all times, in all situations, during all activities, without exception.

AN ASPECT OF INHIBITION

The element of timing characterizes inhibition but does not define it. In other words, it is not sufficient to suspend action for a moment and then go ahead with it in your habitual manner; you will not have changed your action, you will simply have delayed it. You must go beyond waiting before acting and beyond altering the rhythm or speed of an action, and give up the desire to act altogether.

Here is a simple illustration. I put my hands on your head and neck and say, 'Let me turn your head.' It is quite likely that you will then immediately turn your head yourself; indeed, that is how most beginners tend to react to this simple instruction. In this case I would ask you not to react so quickly, and would repeat my request: 'Let me turn your head.' You now have three choices: to turn your head for me as you did before, to prevent me from turning your head by stiffening your neck, or to let your neck be free and allow me to turn your head instead. If you wait a moment and again turn your head, you will not have inhibited your action, but merely delayed it. If you stiffen your neck and prevent me from turning your head, you will have changed your initial reaction, without inhibiting your desire to *do* and to control. It is only by freeing your neck and allowing me to turn your head that you will have inhibited properly.

The first two possible reactions – to do and to block – are both normal. The third reaction – to allow – is natural. To inhibit, then, means both waiting before reacting *and* giving up the wish to react in your normal way.

THE TEACHER'S TOUCH

The teacher touches the pupil for four separate but interrelated reasons. First, touch is an effective way of analysing the pupil's use. Visual observation is an invaluable source of information for an Alexander teacher, yet there are aspects of a pupil's use which are hidden to the teacher's eyes but revealed to the touch of his or her hands.

Second, by touching a pupil, the teacher can help that person prevent certain misuses. For instance, by holding your head and neck in a certain way as you sit and stand, I can prevent you from pulling your head back and down, contracting your neck, and shortening your spine.

Third, at the same time as a teacher prevents a pupil from doing certain things, he or she encourages him to use himself in new and different, inhabitual ways. I described earlier how I may take a pupil off balance, with my hands placed on his shoulders. The position of my hands and my way of using them allow me to point his shoulders outwards, so that they widen instead of contracting.

There are teachers who prefer to guide pupils exclusively through words, arguing that, rather than being given new experiences, the pupil should live *through* them, thereby undertaking the same journey of self-discovery as Alexander. There are also pupils who, for various reasons, do not like being touched by a teacher. Is it possible to learn the principles of the Technique without ever being touched by a teacher's hands?

According to Pablo Casals, the great cellist, '*Si la pensée est juste, tout va*' ('if the thinking is right, everything works'). The ultimate objective of the Alexander Technique is to change your way of thinking. After all, it is a change in attitude and perception that engenders changes in habit, posture, and movement. It should then be possible for you to learn these new habits through a thinking process rather than through touch – possible, but *extremely difficult*, in view of the ever-present gap between what we do and what we think we do. Indeed, the fourth and most important reason why a teacher uses touch is because it can help the pupil to feel more accurately. Thanks to the teacher's touch, the pupil can go through well-conceived and well-directed new experiences, and, from these experiences, draw enough information to overcome the obstacles of faulty sensory awareness and close the gap between what he does and what he feels that he does.

One of my finest pupils is an amateur cellist called Geneviève; we have worked in a steady and rigorous manner for more than six years, and I consider her to be an expert in inhibition and direction. She has learned a great deal about the Technique almost without receiving the touch of my hands, but the absence of my touch has been largely compensated by a number of other factors. Above all, her cello – mirror, guide, companion, source of innumerable problems as well as of constant inspiration – has allowed us to explore every aspect of the Technique. If you are persevering and disciplined, if you have a rich field to explore (such as the cello, or golf, or a martial art), and if you have a resourceful and imaginative teacher, then you too could learn the Alexander Technique without being touched by a teacher's hands. In my view, Geneviève is an exception who only makes the rule all the more relevant.

The overlapping functions of the teacher's hands – 'reading' the pupil's use, preventing misuse, and encouraging good use, all the while helping him feel how he uses himself – are hardly independent of each other. If I put my hands around your ribcage in order to monitor your breathing, the moment I touch you, your attention is naturally drawn to your ribcage and to your breathing. This redirection of your attention inevitably leads to changes in your breathing, however neutral my touch may be.

The teacher uses the hands in a variety of ways. By using hands to guide a pupil through a gesture, the teacher increases a pupil's awareness of his general co-ordination; his enhanced awareness helps him alter and control his use. This *guiding touch* is the mainstay of an Alexander teacher, and it accounts for many of the changes of gesture and thought that a pupil goes through.

Ideally, the teacher should always persuade the pupil to react in a certain way, without forcing him to do so, yet there are times when a pupil is strongly resistant to change. There are many reasons for this, including fear of the unknown, entrenched end-gaining habits, a particular lack of sensorial and kinaesthetic ease, or simply an unwillingness to abandon old controls. By using hands with speed and resolve, a teacher may by-pass a hardy pupil's old controls and give him a new, unexpected experience, which brings with it startling sensations, sometimes of discomfort, sometimes of pleasure. Here, the teacher's touch is *goading* more than guiding. This can be extremely useful, but it takes a skilful teacher to bring it off without harm.

Although the aim of every teacher should be not to treat or cure disease but to teach pupils how to inhibit and direct, the touch of an able teacher may well have soothing and healing properties. A pupil may come in for a lesson suffering from a headache, for example, and leave the lesson forty minutes later free from pain. This often presents a teacher with several dilemmas.

FEELING GOOD, DOING THE RIGHT THING

Pupils who find themselves free from pain after an Alexander lesson may expect the same result after every lesson. However, a moment's freedom cannot ever be reproduced; other moments of perhaps even greater freedom may occur, but not in a predictable or controllable way. The growth of an Alexander pupil almost never follows a straight line in the same forward direction. In an old and wise book we read that 'he who increaseth knowledge increaseth sorrow'. To become newly aware of wrongful habits may make you feel as if the Alexander Technique makes you worse, rather than better. Inevitably, the pupil will go through periods of confusion, discouragement, and frustration.

Also, we tend to confuse the joy of discovering a new thing with the thing itself. The first time you find yourself lengthened and widened as you lie on your back on a teacher's table, you experience great elation – both at being lengthened and widened, and at the novelty of an amazing discovery. The next time around, the sensation is no longer a discovery, and soon you start to take it for granted. The lengthening and widening of your back remain quite real, but the experience may cease to be so intoxicating.

The aim of a teacher is not to make you feel good, but to help you stop doing what is wrong, so that the right thing may do itself.

Touching Others

'I took a number of Alexander lessons. They did me so much good that I would like to share my knowledge of the Technique with my friends and family.'

People who start learning the Alexander Technique are often so amazed at their discovery that they feel a great need to talk about the Technique, to share their experiences, and to preach to others and 'convert' them. To the neophyte, it is obvious that 'the whole world' needs to learn the Technique – every man and woman he sees is misusing himself or herself the whole time – and he is terribly tempted to help others live better. His friends and family ask him about the principles of the Technique and about what goes on during a lesson. As it turns out, the Technique is much easier to demonstrate than to describe or explain. To satisfy the curiosity of his friends as well as his own need to help them, the neophyte finds himself giving little Alexander lessons, in which he tries to imitate the touch of his teacher.

Touching others is an entirely natural impulse. A woman gives her lover a back rub. Two brothers hug each other. A mother holds and cuddles her baby for hours. A young man guides a friend during a workout at the gym. In dozens of situations, touching others is not only natural but needed and welcome. This is not to say that touching others is *always* needed and welcome. There are times when it may be inappropriate, and perhaps even dangerous and harmful.

An Alexander teacher has usually received 1,600 hours or more of professional training, including learning how to use the hands according to a sophisticated and precise method, under the supervision of an experienced director of training. Before ever touching others, the teacher-in-training develops a fine awareness of his or her whole co-ordination, from head to toe. This co-ordination is inseparable from an attitude and a philosophy, which we call *non-doing*. The hands of a trained teacher are certainly very sensitive, yet they play a secondary role in the teacher's co-ordination and pedagogy. It is thanks to this set of aspects – the long and disciplined training, the use of the whole self, attitude and philosophy – that a teacher's hands are soothing, all-knowing, and life-giving.

Almost by definition, the beginner is far from having developed these characteristics. Despite his best intentions, he risks doing harm to a friend when he touches him in an attempt to demonstrate the Alexander Technique. We all suffer from faulty sensory awareness – the ever-present gap between what we do and what we think we do. Our first responsibility before helping others, whether by touching them or by any other means, is to lessen or eliminate this gap in our own use.

The touch of the lover who rubs her partner's back is different from that of the mother who caresses her baby. The touch of an Alexander teacher, too, is different from other touches. The young mother who studies the Technique may well learn to touch her baby with a mixture of firmness and suppleness that the baby will find reassuring and agreeable. All the same, she will always touch her baby as a mother, not as an Alexander teacher. When you touch a friend, a child, even a cat or a dog, you should do it with intelligence and sensitivity. However, you should never allow yourself to take the rôle of an amateur Alexander teacher by touching others as if giving them an Alexander lesson.

Touching Others continued

To proselytize for something difficult to describe and explain is an enormous challenge. Some would claim, with good reason, that to *proselytize non-doing* is a contradiction in terms. If you wish to make the Alexander Technique better known, there are several possibilities that do not involve your using your hands. Invite interested parties to watch some of the lessons you are taking yourself from a qualified teacher; invite them to share a lesson; offer to pay for a lesson as a birthday gift; or encourage them to read articles or books about the Technique.

The desire to help others sometimes hides a desire to change or to control them. Our first duty is to change ourselves, and to let others change themselves, when they are ready to change, and if they want to change. Non-doing applies to all aspects of life, including interpersonal relationships. Often the best way, and sometimes the only way, to help someone else is to *do nothing* – above all, to do nothing that may aggravate the state of the person in question or the state of your relationship with him or her (*see* Chapter 5).

Finally, you may help and influence your family, friends, and colleagues indirectly, by becoming a model of good use, clear thinking, and comportment that is not end-gaining. If you use yourself well, are confident of your good use, and remain faithful to the principles and practices of the Alexander Technique, people around you will be encouraged to imitate you and to learn from you.

Sometimes, the right thing feels very good indeed. At other times, to act against comfortable habits requires sacrifice, self-restraint, and a disciplined will. Before you master it, 'thinking up' may be awkward and even painful. Therefore, both teacher and pupil should regard the intoxicating moments of release, pleasure, and freedom experienced in an Alexander lesson with equal gratitude and circumspection.

Since an Alexander teacher uses his or her hands, it is tempting for the layman to compare the Technique with other hands-on methods such as massage, acupressure, osteopathy or chiropractic. There may well be points of contact between these various disciplines, which all have their own merits, yet the touch of an Alexander teacher has individual properties, a consequence of both the aims and methods of the Technique. Some of these properties are difficult to describe, and are best experienced personally.

Once you have felt the touch of an Alexander teacher, you run the risk of experiencing certain feelings (*see* box on 'Touching Others').

TRADITIONAL PROCEDURES

In order to learn the Technique, all you need is a stimulus that triggers a reaction. Your reaction is most likely to be normal. If you then inhibit it and direct your use, you may pass from normal to natural. The stimulus itself is not important; sitting and standing, walking, juggling, speaking, and many other activities are perfectly suited to the task.

In his teaching practice, Alexander used certain specific procedures, which he had created or adapted. It seems appropriate to end this chapter with a description of some of these procedures. I have chosen the monkey, the lunge, the whispered 'ah', and constructive rest, and will describe them only briefly.

The reason for this is that it is nearly impossible to learn how to do something well from a written description. Most people would agree that even an excellent book about singing would not be sufficient for a reader who has never sung to learn how to use his voice, however resourceful that reader may be. The descriptions that follow are not meant to teach you how to perform these procedures by yourself; rather, they are intended to arouse your curiosity and imagination.

The Monkey

When a good tennis player hits a backhand across the court, she bends her knees and leans forward from the hips, using her back and legs in an active and dynamic manner. Her spinal column is firm and elastic, and the articulations throughout her body – hips, knees, and ankles – are perfectly free. Her head is poised on top of her spine, and moves independently from the trunk as she follows the ball with her eyes. This position gives the player great stability and mobility; she can alter her position with ease and speed, and as she moves on the court she never loses her balance, even when she runs, comes to a sudden halt, or changes direction.

The golfer, the dancer, and the small child who lowers himself to pick up a toy all use this position. Indeed, it is a good way to lower your body – to sit down, to brush your teeth, to take a drink of water from a fountain, to pick up a heavy object – without sacrificing its length. Alexander used to refer to this position, among others, as a 'position of mechanical advantage'. His students preferred the more evocative name of 'the monkey'.

The first time an Alexander teacher helps you into this position, you are likely to react 'normally', with all that this implies; you will end-gain and misuse your whole self while experiencing feelings of unbalance and

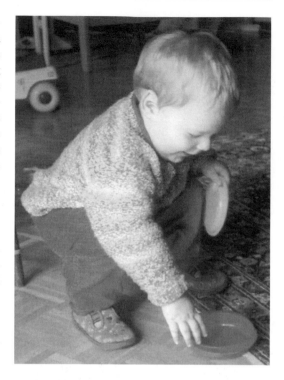

uneasiness. You will find it difficult to believe that the monkey is a natural position. The monkey is, therefore, an invaluable laboratory of self-awareness, which deals with issues of tension, relaxation, effort, co-ordination, balance, strength, inhibition and direction, besides being a position that has great usefulness in daily life.

The Lunge

The lunge is another fine method of considering the differences between what is normal and what is natural. It is similar to the monkey in the way that it requires the organized use of the back and legs. People who are well co-ordinated – dancers, martial artists, sportsmen and women, children at play – go in and out of lunges constantly in their daily lives, whether consciously or by reflex, instinctively or intuitively.

When you lunge, your head is perfectly balanced on top of the spine, your neck is neither contracted nor floppy, and your body is pointed upwards, stable and dynamic. One foot rests slightly forward of the other and is turned a little outwards; the front leg is bent and the back one straight, but both are ready to bend or unbend as necessary, in alternation or simultaneously, as dictated by need or desire. Typified by a fencer at play, the lunge is useful as an all-purpose standing position, when pushing a heavy door open, or for a flautist or a violinist performing a concerto.

The lunge is not a rigid posture; on the contrary, the body retains its mobility at all times. It is possible, and easy, to alter its many variables: the distance and angle between the feet, the degree of bending of the various joints (hips, knees, and ankles), and the position of the trunk or of the head. If you place yourself in a close-footed lunge, you will be able to stand for longer without tiring your back than with your feet parallel to each other, as you are less likely to let your pelvis sink forward or to hollow your lower back.

Note that it is easy to go from a monkey into a lunge and vice-versa, to sit down or to squat from a monkey, to start walking from a lunge, and to stop walking and place yourself in a lunge. A well co-ordinated person should find it comfortable to go from one gesture to the other, so that doing a monkey or a lunge, squatting, sitting, standing, and walking all spring one from the other in a fluid, continuous line of thought and movement.

No position is good in itself; it becomes good or bad, health-giving or harmful, according to the way you direct yourself into

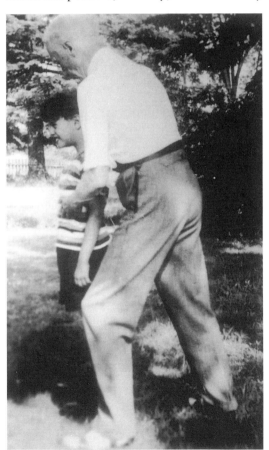

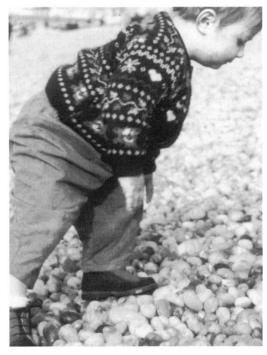

the position, within it, and out of it. These directions – the chief of which is 'thinking up along the spine' – are impossible to describe; even if it were possible to describe them with the utmost precision, you would find it difficult to put them into practice without the guidance of an experienced observer.

Useful as they may be in daily life, the monkey and the lunge are means much more than ends. Doing ten monkeys in a row would do you little good. However, using the monkey to find out about faulty sensory awareness, end-gaining, inhibition and direction, the Primary Control, and the passing from normal to natural would be the best thing you could do for your well-being.

The Whispered 'Ah'

The late writer, teacher and visionary Sir George Trevelyan was on Alexander's first training course in the 1930s. He wrote in his diary, 'Asked what he considered the essential way for a sedentary worker to keep in condition, F. M. said without hesitation: "The whispered 'ah', particularly over the chair."'[8]

The whispered 'ah' is much more than a way for a sedentary person to keep in condition. It is a formidable psychomotor challenge, rich in opportunities for inhibiting and directing. Find your Primary Directions: 'Let the neck be free, to let the head go forward and up, to let the back lengthen and widen, all together, one after the other.' Carry on thinking up along the spine, and smile (thus opening your nostrils and sinuses, and lifting your soft palate). Carry on thinking up and smiling, and direct your jaw slightly forward (to prevent it from cramming into your skull or down on to the throat). Carry on thinking up, smiling, and directing your jaw forward, and open your mouth, without letting your tongue contract backwards. Carry on thinking up, smiling, directing your jaw forward, opening your mouth and leaving your tongue relaxed, and let your lungs empty themselves as you emit the vowel 'ah' in a stage whisper. Carry on thinking up, close your mouth without retracting your jaw backwards, let air enter your lungs through your nose, and release your smile.

I offer this description of the whispered 'ah' in the absolute certainty that you will be unable to perform it correctly. Indeed, my description is not meant to lead you through a whispered 'ah', but to help you imagine how complex and all-encompassing a procedure it is. It demands the capacity to give multiple directions in a well-defined hierarchy, which is in itself a difficult thing to do; and it demands that you 'think up' first and foremost, which is something that you cannot learn from a book.

Every beginner who struggles with the whispered 'ah' for the first time end-gains and misuses himself or herself to a remarkable degree. The reverse of the coin, logically, is that someone who has mastered the whispered 'ah' has mastered his or her use. The whispered 'ah' requires the co-ordination of the whole body, a supple and firm spine, a free neck and a mobile head, the harmonious use of the mechanisms of the lips, tongue, and jaw, the perfect balance of the torso, an elastic ribcage, the free use of the voice, and much more.

The whispered 'ah' may be used in preparation for speech, to improve enunciation, to open and clean the sinuses, and as complementary therapy in treating Temporal-Mandibular Syndrome and other dental and skeletal problems related to the co-ordination of the jaw. Well-executed whispered 'ah's have a double effect, of energizing and calming at the same time, and can help mitigate stage fright and moments of stress and agitation. People have used it to stop an attack of hiccups, to ward off the onset of migraine, and to deal with the effects of air pressure when landing and taking off in an plane. My teacher, the late Patrick

Macdonald, claimed that it was also useful in dealing with hangovers.

The whispered 'ah' opens a door into the world of breathing. Alexander saw breathing is a function of co-ordination. Everyone whose breathing is imperfect is badly co-ordinated; indeed, the very imperfections of co-ordination create the imperfections in breathing. If you wish to breathe perfectly, all you need to do is to co-ordinate yourself, leaving your breathing to right itself. According to Alexander, the control of breathing should happen only indirectly, which puts the Technique in frontal opposition with all methods of direct control of breathing.

'The act of breathing', he wrote, 'is not a primary, or even a secondary, part of the process ... As a matter of fact, given the perfect co-ordination of parts as required by my system, breathing is a subordinate operation which will perform itself.[9]... *It is not necessary ... even to think of taking a breath; as a matter of fact, it is more or less harmful to do so.*'[10]

The whispered 'ah', then, is not a breathing exercise in the way that most people conceive of breathing exercises, but, rather, an exercise in co-ordination. Your co-ordination is synonymous with the use you make of yourself as you react to a given stimulus. Explore the whispered 'ah' not to improve or control your breathing, but to become aware of the way you use yourself and of all the many consequences your use has upon your breathing.

One last remark about the whispered 'ah': according to Alexander, and as illustrated by the way the whispered 'ah' is constructed, the breathing cycle starts with an expiration, followed by an inspiration. If you co-ordinate yourself well as you let air out of your lungs, the subsequent intake of breath should be a simple reflex, not an act of the conscious will. Think about this next time you decide to 'take a deep breath'.

Constructive Rest

We arrive finally at a point of rest. Imagine a long and difficult day – you may have had a contentious family visit, a looming deadline at the office, or a commute in heavy traffic. Imagine that, right in the middle of the afternoon of such a day, you have an irresistible need to get a little rest. You lie down on your bed or on a couch, and you fall asleep briefly, your body more or less folded on itself, your arms tightly crossed in front of your chest, your shoulders raised, your mind still preoccupied with the difficulties of the day. You wake up after a few moments, more anxious and tense and fatigued than before.

Now imagine a different way of resting in the middle of a demanding day. You lie down comfortably on your bed, and fall asleep quickly and deeply. When you wake up forty minutes later, you feel heavy and slow, and you spend the rest of the day yawning, hankering for some coffee, and yearning to return to the delights of sleep and oblivion.

Often the best way to deal with fatigue is to rest until the fatigue is no more. This may require a long night's sleep or a week by the seaside, yet the requirements of daily living, of work and family, do not always permit this. In the absence of ideal rest, it may be better to avoid taking a quick nap that leaves you tense and anxious, or a longer rest that leaves you heavy and lethargic. Instead, you may opt for a moment of *constructive rest*, in which calm, quietude, and good co-ordination help you regain a measure of energy and alertness.

In an Alexander lesson, the teacher asks you to lie down on a table covered with a couple of folded blankets or another material that softens the surface of the table. The teacher guides you into a position known to all Alexandrians: on your back, your legs bent at the knees, the soles of your feet down on the table, your arms pronated (that is, the palms of your hands facing downwards), your elbows bent, and your hands placed on your abdomen. Your head rests on a support – a small pillow, a folded towel or one or two books. Without this support, your head would fall backwards and down, exaggerating the curve of your neck, shortening your spine, and constricting your throat.

The teacher stretches your back while respecting the natural curves of your spine, by lifting and tilting your pelvis and then placing it just a little further down the table, or by placing his or her hands under your upper back and scooping it upwards and outwards. In this position, your body is stretched, lengthened, widened, supported, and released. During the lesson the teacher takes advantage of this position and the inner state that accompanies it to work on various parts of your body, bringing your attention to a limb, a set of muscles, your neck, your ribcage, and helping you become aware of how you use or misuse yourself. The teacher may ask you to move a limb without disturbing the arrangement of the head and neck, or to speak a vowel or a word without shortening your neck or narrowing your back,

or to perform a few whispered 'ah's. In sum, he or she helps you inhibit and direct. After a while you are guided off the table, and you feel calm, strong, open, and centred.

Needless to say, your teacher shows you how to place yourself in this position, how to stretch your own back, and how to gauge the support needed by your head and neck. After you learn how to rest constructively, you get into the habit of spending a few minutes, at home or in the office, in such a state of co-ordination, remaining alert and responsive, becoming ever more aware of your use, savouring the upward thought in your spine, and inhibiting and directing. In time you will feel as strong and calm when you work on yourself at home as when you leave your teacher's table.

You may lie on your back to listen to the radio or to have a long phone conversation with a friend, to think or to meditate, to memorize some text or a page of music for a concert you must give, to calm yourself after a moment of stress or conflict, and above all to sharpen your capacity to inhibit and direct – the ultimate goal of every procedure of the Alexander Technique.

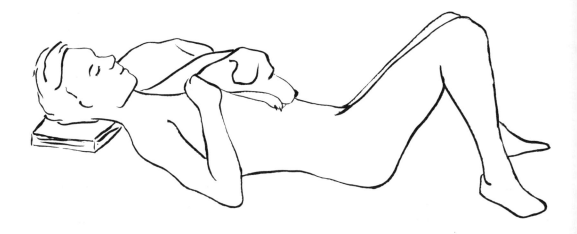

CHAPTER 5
Emotions

BODY AND MIND

Most people believe that the interaction between body and mind goes like this: I perceive something – an event, a person, a sensation; this perception gives me an emotion – joy, anger, fear; this in turn affects my physical state – my breathing changes, my circulation speeds up, my legs start to shake.

This chain of events implies a degree of separation between body and mind, however close the interaction between them may be. After all, it states that the mind reacts to something before the body does. Further, it seems to place the burden of our emotions upon the mind: our bodily reactions are just a side-effect of our mind's perceptions.

William James, considered by many to be the father of modern psychology, proposed an alternative to this understanding: I perceive something – an event, a person, a sensation; this perception immediately affects my physical state – my breathing changes, my circulation speeds up, my legs start to shake. In James's words, 'the bodily changes follow directly from the perception of the exciting fact and ... our feeling of the same changes as they occur *is* the emotion'[11] – joy, anger, fear.

In a recent newspaper article, we find James's century-old views curiously validated. Current neurobiological research argues that 'emotions and feelings are not, as poets and philosophers say, ephemeral reflections of the human soul', but, rather, 'the brain's interpretation of our visceral reaction to the world at large'.[12] Jorge Luis Borges, paraphrasing Coleridge, wrote that, in our dreams, 'images represent the sensations we think they cause; we do not feel horror because we are threatened by a sphinx; we dream of a sphinx in order to explain the horror we feel.'[13] Let us turn this insight into a general statement. We do not experience a physical sensation to express this or that emotion; we use the vocabulary of emotions to speak of this or that physical state.

It is impossible, then, to separate emotions from bodily states. Imagine a strong emotion – anger, for example, or elation. Picture the physical sensations that you associate with the emotion. Now try to picture the same emotion without its physical sensations. Quite simply, the emotion ceases to exist.

The Alexander Technique confirms and enriches James's view of the relationship between emotions and bodily states. First, the Technique alters our sensory awareness. By making it more objective and reliable, it changes the perceptions we have of the world and of ourselves, and the way we process these perceptions. Since our perceptions condition our reactions, to see the world in a different light is to react differently to it, and to live differently in it. Following James's argument, our new perceptions lead directly to bodily states that are necessarily different from those we used to have when we saw the world in the old

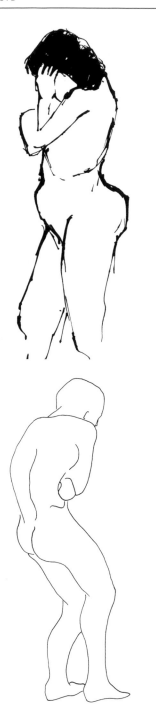

Is distress a mental state or a physical one?

light. Since bodily states are emotions themselves, changing our perceptions inevitably leads to change in our emotions.

PERCEPTIONS AND REACTIONS

As well as changing the way we perceive the world, the Technique also affects the interplay between our perceptions and the reactions that they engender. For most people, every perception leads automatically to a more or less pre-set (that is, habitual) reaction. The person who reacts in this way is often unaware of the reaction taking place, and of its quality as a bodily reality and emotion.

The Alexander Technique helps you break down the automatic link between perception and reaction, so that you do not necessarily and inevitably react to everything you perceive. Alexandrian inhibition makes it possible for you to wait before reacting, and to choose your reaction. It also enlarges your range of possible reactions. In this way you react according to the needs of each situation, instead of reacting like a mouse in a laboratory maze. The greatest benefit of this approach is that it allows you *not to react at all*, if you so desire or if the situation does not warrant a reaction from you.

The effects of this on your emotions should be evident. Thanks to inhibition, you will become able to respond differently to situations or to people who normally evoke strong or unpleasant emotions. You may have said of somebody, 'He irritates me.' It would be more accurate and useful to say, 'I am irritated by him.' Better still would be, 'I allow myself to be automatically irritated by him.' With the help of the Alexander Technique, you may one day say, 'I do not need to react to him, and if I do it is only because I want to.'

Alexander pupils often go through a revolution when they understand for the first time in their life that they are responsible for the way they react to people or to events. Having blamed an in-law for a conflict for many years, they may suddenly realize that it is their automatic, habitual, pre-set and unaware reaction to the in-law that causes the problem. Their in-law reacts differently to them if they react differently to him or her. This in turn dissipates the conflict and allows the two people to relate to each other differently on a permanent

---

Alexis, 28, Artist

Before the Alexander Technique I thought that it might cure my persistent lower back pain. Since I started lessons I have discovered many benefits, only one of which is a better understanding of how to use my back.

Before the Alexander Technique I used to think that it was comfortable to slide down in my chair, legs crossed in front of me, arms across my chest, head hanging down. Now I think I need to change my furniture to accommodate my upward thinking.

Before the Alexander Technique I used to walk with my head down, looking at my feet. After the Alexander Technique I discovered that eye contact is not fatal – a lesson I am still digesting.

Before the Alexander Technique I used to catch glimpses of myself in the mirror that could ruin my entire day. Now I catch glimpses of myself in mirrors that please me.

Before the Alexander Technique, exercising and eating healthy foods were things I had to force myself to do. Now exercising and eating well have become effortlessly easier. I feel in control of my body for the first time in my life, and take pleasure in it.

Before the Alexander Technique, if something was not right in my life it would overwhelm me and permeate other areas of my life. After the Alexander Technique something can be terribly wrong, but I can still be fundamentally happy.

Before the Alexander Technique I did not like to be alone very much. After the Alexander Technique I have discovered that I like my time alone. I am perfectly capable of finding fun and interesting things to do by myself.

Before the Alexander Technique I had fixed ideas about myself. Since the Alexander Technique I find I am frequently surprised by my feelings and actions.

Before the Alexander Technique I was content to 'go with the flow', to see where life led. Since the Alexander Technique I desire to have more input in my life. I have discovered that I am ambitious.

Before the Alexander Technique I thought I had figured out some things about life. Now I realize I am not as smart as I thought I was.

Before the Alexander Technique I was more judgmental of myself and others. Now I surprise myself by wanting to break rules.

Before the Alexander Technique I thought being selfish was the worst thing one could be. I would try to hide my selfish desires. Now I express them more readily and admire others who do, too.

Before the Alexander Technique, my emotions were usually steady. Now I experience intense emotions – intense sadness as well as intense joy. I express my feelings more easily. I laugh more heartily if not necessarily more often.

basis. (For further discussion of interpersonal relationships, *see* later in the chapter.)

People often justify their behaviour by saying, 'That is just the way I am,' or 'It is stronger than me,' or 'There is nothing I can do about it.' This is a way of washing their hands of the consequences of their actions, as it implies that they are incapable of reacting in any way other than their habitual one. Such an attitude has grave moral and social repercussions; as an explanation or justification for objectionable behaviour, it is plainly untenable.

If you have never considered the link between your perceptions and your automatic reactions, you may feel justified in your belief that others *make* you react the way you do, or that your reaction is the only possible one. All the same, until you become capable of *not reacting at will, and in every conceivable situation*, and unless you have experienced the possibilities of reaction that follow from this capacity, you cannot say that your true nature is reflected in the person that you are today. Think about it. If your reactions are automatic and habitual, and if you are not even aware of your behaviours and of the mechanisms that animate them, then you are no more than a bundle of reflexes and instincts, just like an insect or a reptile. Is this your true nature?

To be true to yourself implies making choices. The freedom to choose is an innate ability of every human being; indeed, it defines the human species. Yet, like many other human attributes, its flowering requires constant care and cultivation. To become free to choose – which means above all *to be free from the lack of choice* – is a lifelong struggle for most people. By reacting immediately and automatically to every stimulation, you eliminate even the possibility of choice. Therefore, you need first to learn how *not* to react before you can claim to having made a choice. Then, and only then, will your actions reflect your true nature.

To be able to choose does not imply the ability consistently to make good choices. To do the right thing often requires courage, sacrifice, and self-restraint, all of which often fail us. However, the person who understands that his or her actions are the result of a series of choices is better able to handle the consequences of his or her choices, poor as they may be. To say, 'I made an error of judgement,' or 'I allowed myself some short-term satisfaction despite the price I paid in the long term,' is a much more constructive statement than, 'It was his fault,' or 'That is who I am.'

The Alexander Technique is not the only method of dealing with your choices and the emotions that animate them and that are in turn fed by them. It does not matter how you acquire the twin abilities not to react and to choose your reactions, but you will not be a free, healthy, and happy person until you do so.

THE RATIONAL AND THE IRRATIONAL

One of the arguments sometimes put forward against Alexandrian inhibition is that it leads the rational to over-dominate the creative, the imaginative, and the intuitive, causing a loss of spontaneity, or a loss of freedom. It would be useful here to define 'freedom', so that we can understand 'spontaneity' better.

Many people equate freedom with the possibility of doing whatever they feel like, regardless of circumstances. The range of behaviours some of these people allow themselves may be more or less narrow, but the principle is the same: 'I want to do this, or to be this way, and, unless I am allowed to, I am not free.' However, if your wants are predetermined – if your reactions are habitual and automatic, and if you are not aware of your reactions or of their motivations – then you are not free, even if you allow yourself all that you would ever want. In truth, you will not know what your real needs are before you can exercise complete restraint, particularly over the wish to satisfy every desire the moment the desire manifests itself.

This is not a puritanical or ascetic view. Alexandrians drink, smoke, dance, take recreational drugs and make love in the back seat of cars. It is *not being able to do otherwise* that is a problem. If you have the capacity to choose, you are a free person. If you do not, you are not, however good it feels to indulge yourself. To be spontaneous means making a choice that is unencumbered by preconceived ideas and assumptions. If your choice is influenced by habit or addiction, then you are not spontaneous.

In this matter some people make an intellectual headstand, and proclaim that they *wish* to be addicted – to sugar, alcohol, nicotine or other chemical substances, or to a thought pattern or behaviour. This is pure sophistry and not worthy of discussion. Surely everyone would agree that true freedom and spontaneity flow from choice, not from habit.

Interestingly, studies have shown that young children who can exercise self-restraint – for instance, agreeing to accept two sweets after a few moments rather than consuming one immediately – are much more likely to succeed later in life, both personally and professionally. Self-restraint, then, leads to an increase in well-being. (This is one of the points made by Daniel Goleman in his book *Emotional Intelligence*, which offers many intriguing insights for students of Alexandrian inhibition.)

So, some people claim (or fear) that Alexandrian inhibition stifles creativity. Reason and creativity are not mutually exclusive attributes; on the contrary. Some people are said to be 'too rational', but if you observe their behaviours closely, you will start seeing how deeply irrational the *motivations* for those behaviours really are. To give a trivial example: if someone decides always to wear the same kind of clothes – white shirt, grey trousers, black shoes, for example – life will be easier (he will not have to worry about picking what to buy or what to wear), but is his decision rational? It is practical, maybe, but not rational. It denotes a fear of variety, a failure of the healthy grooming instinct, perhaps even a suppression of sensuality and sexuality. To my mind, these factors make the behaviour in question *irrational*. It is almost impossible for someone to be too rational. Often, however, the interplay of the rational and the irrational is unbalanced.

At times, people claim that a belief or behaviour of theirs is rational, in order to justify it. It is possible to convince yourself *and* others of the rationality of an irrational belief, through power of personality or persuasive discourse. Not long ago, millions of people believed that the extermination of Jews, Gypsies, and homosexuals could be rationally justified and rationally accomplished. This is an extreme example, but it illustrates forcefully the enormous gap that exists between rationality and intellectually argued irrationality. This gap is evident in thousands of beliefs and behaviours in politics, science, religion, art – in fact, in every conceivable situation.

Indeed, we all adhere to a number of irrational beliefs, completely innocent of their irrationality. It is our duty to become aware of the underlying irrationality of these beliefs, and of the effects they have upon the way we relate to other people, and upon our health and well-being. Then, of course, we need to change or eliminate these beliefs, *whenever they are harmful* (which is not necessarily always).

It is amazing how many people believe in something simply because somebody else also believes in it. Alexander was fond of saying, 'I believe in everything, and I believe in nothing.' This is the ultimate statement of open-mindedness. It says that it does not matter how many people believe in something, or how famous some of these people may be; if it is demonstrably false, I will not believe in it. It does not matter how few people believe in something, or how humble some of these people may be; if it is demonstrably true, I will believe in it. Somebody may have been consistently right over a period of time; I will not suppose that he is *always* right. I will apply the same principle for somebody who has been wrong many times. I may detest a certain woman, but if what she says is right, I cannot possibly deny it. If a madman says that Paris is the capital of France, he is mad, but he is right. 'I believe in everything, and I believe in nothing.'

Every cherished opinion, however sincerely held, should be liable to impartial scrutiny. For your scrutiny to be of any value, however, your perceptions need to be clear and accurate. Your capacity to discern and judge is a direct function of your sensory awareness. 'We have to recognize,' wrote Alexander, 'that our sensory peculiarities are the foundation of what we think of as our opinions, and that, in fact, nine out of ten of the opinions we form are rather the result of what we feel than what we think.'[14] I have explained elsewhere the relationship that exists between the use of the self and sensory awareness. Your self is the instrument through which you observe and perceive. If you misuse yourself, your observations and perceptions will be distorted by faulty sensory awareness. Your opinions and beliefs derived from these distorted perceptions will then be distorted too, and, consequently, invalid. Alexander used to say that 'it doesn't alter a fact because you can't feel it'.[15] We can expand the dictum to say that a fact does not become a fact simply because you 'feel' it.

Getting rid of beliefs based on faulty perceptions – 'facts' which do not exist outside your perceptions – would by definition make you more rational. Yet your creativity need not be diminished in any way. The aim of the Alexander Technique is not for the conscious will to dominate the subconscious, nor for the rational to supplant the irrational. Every person will always remain an admixture of these contrasting forces; it is hardly possible for things to be otherwise. However, it is possible to change the way the two forces interact, so that the irrational becomes a healthy source of intuition, creativity, imagination, insight, and humour. 'As a matter of fact,' Alexander said, 'feeling is much more use than what they call "mind" when it is right.'[16] Here, Alexander leaves implicit the difference between reason and intellectually argued irrationality, which is often confused with 'mind'. (I suspect that by 'they', Alexander meant intellectuals and academics. In Alexander's circle of friends and students, a 'Nobel prize' was a derogatory epithet reserved for a seemingly intelligent person who said or did particularly inept things.) Reason and feeling are not contradictory. On the contrary; since feeling is the source of all observation, and observation the source of reason, it is feeling that gives reason its inherent rightness, *as long as feeling itself is free from imprecision or distortion.*

INHIBITION AND THE EXPRESSION OF FEELINGS

Another argument sometimes put forward against Alexandrian inhibition concerns the possible repression of feelings. 'It is unnatural and unhealthy not to feel, not to express these genuinely felt emotions, and not to act upon them,' the argument goes. As with every other argument, context and circumstance may render the argument partially or wholly invalid, valid sometimes but not always, right for the wrong reasons, or wrong for the right reasons. It all depends.

(In passing, note that the word 'inhibition' has connotations that make it difficult for some people to accept it as a beneficial force. This is unfortunate, for, in the context of the Technique, 'inhibition' is a perfectly good word to use to refer to the ability not to react habitually and automatically.)

It may be useful for us to establish a difference between acting and reacting. Freedom means the capacity to choose your reactions. This includes the choice *not to react*, if the situation does not merit a reaction or if you simply wish not to react. If your reactions flow from this capacity, they *become* actions. If not, they *remain* reactions, closer in nature to animal reflexes than to positive acts of an individual will.

For a person who has not yet acquired the capacity not to react automatically and habitually to every stimulus, the suppression of emotion or of its expression may be harmful. It has long been thought that suppressed emotion is an important factor in the onset and development of a host of serious diseases, including ulcers, heart attacks, breathing disorders, apoplexy, cancer, and so on. This opinion is widely but not universally held. Some psychologists maintain that expressing all emotions freely is not necessarily healthier than not expressing them. Dr Mark Epstein, psychiatrist and author of *Thoughts without a Thinker*, points out that 'the vent to rage… typically pumps up the brain's arousal, leaving people more angry, not less.'[17] He suggests that it is possible, and desirable, neither to give vent to anger nor to suppress it, but rather to *acknowledge* it; it is better not to react too soon or too strongly.

Becoming free of *automatic and habitual* strong emotions is healthier than feeling and expressing strong emotions. You may not even be aware of these emotions, and they may be unwarranted by the situation or person that elicits them from you; in sum, they are emotions that harm you (and others), whether you express them or not.

Because of faulty sensory awareness, many emotions, both positive and negative, result simply from misreading a situation. You feel slighted or insulted by a nod, a wink or a word from somebody else; you act upon the slight by brooding, or fighting. Yet the nod was not directed at you, and the wink was actually an attempt to shoo away a fly. As for words, they are consistently mis-stated, misheard, and misinterpreted. Sociolinguists have demonstrated that people use such distinct styles to communicate that we all have to 'translate' what others say before understanding them. Alexandrian inhibition allows you to listen, translate, and understand what you hear before reacting to it. The better you use yourself, the more accurately you gauge a situation. Inhibition then allows you to react according to this precise gauging, rather than according to preconceived ideas or habitual patterns of thought and behaviour. If you find a situation difficult to gauge or comprehend, inhibition is again useful, helping you to learn not to react blindly or haphazardly.

The end result of a committed study of the Alexander Technique, then, is not the forceful repression of emotions, but a real change in their quality, intensity, and expression. Pupils often speak of certain things becoming less important. 'Detachment' is the somewhat jaded word that best describes their newly found state of being. Note that I do not speak of an 'inner state', or a 'state of mind'. Let us reaffirm yet again the inseparability of body and mind. The old saying, *mens sana in corpore sano* ('a healthy body is a healthy mind') is redundant: in fact, the one cannot exist without the other.

DETACHMENT

Many passionate and sincere people confuse detachment with a lack of compassion. They believe it to be morally wrong not to do their best in a given situation, and therefore resist the very idea of not reacting. Yet, not to react – that is, not to end-gain, or not to react in an automatic and habitual way – often means doing the very best that a situation or person requires.

My late mother, who smoked two packets of cigarettes a day for nearly forty years, was diagnosed as having lung cancer several years ago. She had always resisted the family's attempts to get her to stop smoking. We tried everything, from reasoning and pleading to emotional blackmail. She would just laugh and light up another cigarette. The onset of her disease made our efforts more insistent but no more efficient. Little by little, I realized that there was nothing any of us could do to make her give up her habit – in other words, there was nothing we could do to *change her*. For a while after I arrived at this understanding, I still wanted to ask her to stop smoking, but I did not say anything. Finally, almost without noticing it, I altogether stopped wanting to make her change, and I accepted her fully – for who she was, as she was. I stopped pleading or hectoring; all I gave her was my quiet affection and support in all her choices, and in her continuing addiction. To some, my detachment in the face of her self-destructive behaviour – my *not reacting* to it – appeared like indifference, cynicism, or even fatalism. '*Do* something!', indignant friends would beseech me. My mother saw my 'indifference' otherwise, and once paid me a great compliment. 'You're not like the others,' she said with gratitude. (My indignant friends, I note in passing, behaved towards me in the way my family had behaved towards my mother, trying to change what could not, and perhaps should not, change.)

After your Alexander training you will still be angered, but perhaps less often and less intensely than before, and by different things and people from before. You may express your anger differently too. Recently, during a working trip to Switzerland, I found myself in a foul mood. I had wanted to go for a walk in the forest, and instead I ended up going on a long and tiring car journey with my travelling companion. That is, I had not got what I wanted and I was quite displeased with the outcome of the situation. Nevertheless, instead of sulking or being irritated, I teased my friend with a series of insults. I was vulgar and aggressive, but also imaginative and humorous. We both laughed, and I managed to let out disagreeable and ultimately unwanted feelings. My bad mood dissipated, simply because I indulged it with creativity.

Alexander teachers like to say that to inhibit means to say 'no' to a habitual reaction, which helps you deal well with difficult situations. But to inhibit also means to say 'no' to a whole situation (rather than to your reaction to it) – for example, to an invitation, a provocation, a temptation, to somebody who wants to tango. When you stop entering conflicts, the whole quality of your emotional life changes. Still, the richer of the two possibilities is not avoiding a situation or eliminating a stimulus, but changing your habitual reaction to it.

THE DISCOMFORT OF CHANGE

All change, however beneficial, and regardless of how it comes about, can be difficult. The emotional changes that the Technique may make in your life are no exception. One personal story illustrates this point very well.

In 1977, when I was nineteen, I left Brazil to go to study the cello in the United States. It was my first time away from home, and I used to write long and detailed letters to my family. My mother kept all my letters, and many years later I put them in chronological order and re-read them. My first year in the USA was a time of intense discovery.

Although I was often homesick and lonely, the overall tone of my letters was one of enthusiasm and excitement. I was fascinated by New York and by the endless contrasts I perceived between my new surroundings and the city where I had grown up. The school I was attending had been founded recently by an idealistic governor who endowed it with magnificent facilities. I thought many of my teachers were brilliant, and my colleagues talented and accomplished. I was a devoted and disciplined student, and was in love with learning and making music.

The letters from my second year tell a starkly different story. I felt that Americans my age were immature and thoughtless. The physical setting of the school was unpleasant and unwelcoming, and the music department badly run. I did not like the food I had to eat. The weather was dreadful. I dreamed of finding another school in a different country – Czechoslovakia, perhaps, or Holland. I had doubts about *myself*, and was filled with self-loathing.

What had happened? Partly these were the natural and inevitable pains of becoming an adult. However, re-reading my letters seventeen years later, I realized that there was a cause and effect relationship between my distress and a new element that had entered my life.

I changed cello teachers at the beginning of my second year of studies. My new teacher felt that my playing would improve if I took some lessons in the Alexander Technique, as I seemed to be somewhat awkward, physically, at the cello. I had heard a little bit about the Technique from other musicians, who always found it difficult to describe but who spoke enthusiastically of its effects on their music-making and on other aspects of their life. I agreed at once to see an Alexander teacher, and made an appointment with someone my cello teacher recommended. She was an older woman who lived in a beautiful apartment on Central Park West. She had been an Alexander

teacher for a few years, and had a maternal presence that I found instantly reassuring.

The very first time she put her hands on my head and neck, I felt myself 'growing' several inches. Under my teacher's hands I felt like one of those flowers we sometimes see on television, where the flower's slow growth has been speeded up so that it takes just a few seconds from planting to full blossoming. It was a delightful sensation, unlike anything I had ever experienced before, and it made me laugh out loud. There were many other strong impressions in this lesson, and in subsequent ones, but my first experience of the Alexander Technique, which has remained with me ever since, was that it was a gift of life.

From early on, the lessons had a profound effect on me. People who did not even know that I was taking Alexander lessons remarked that I looked taller and broader. My shirts and sweaters soon became too tight around the shoulders. There were many other effects, but at the time I found it difficult to pinpoint them. I knew I was changing, but I could not tell what these changes were and how they manifested themselves. I wrote excited letters to my family. I explained to them after my first lesson that the Technique was a mixture of 'relaxation' and 'self-suggestion', using two terms that I would definitely not use today. I told them how wonderful my teacher was, how much I enjoyed her lessons, and how light and alive I felt walking out of her teaching studio.

Yet it was during this same period that I started feeling strongly negative about my school, my teachers, my colleagues, and myself. How could I be receiving a gift of life from a wonderful woman, and feeling worse outside my lessons?

Indeed, it was this very gift that made me miserable. There are many reasons for this. In my Alexander lessons, I moved towards some sort of ideal state of being, free from discomfort, pain, anger, fear, doubt or hesitation. This state did not last long, and, after a day or two – sometimes after just a few hours – I would find myself back where I was before I had ever taken a lesson, without knowing how this deterioration had taken place, how to prevent it, or how to reverse it once it hit me. The contrast between my new Alexander state and my old, usual state seemed enormous. Suddenly, now that I had a taste of an ideal and of the possibilities it presented me, *not to be ideal* was unbearable, hence my self-loathing.

The Alexander ideal I was experiencing went beyond the confines of my being. After all, my teacher was a marvellous woman and our lessons together seemed a perfect human interaction, full of discoveries and adventures, and animated by understanding, insight, and loving support. Why could all my interactions not be like that? Everybody else in the world deviated much too sharply from the Alexander ideal, without even knowing that this ideal existed and how far they were from attaining it. Living in the non-Alexander world was too painful. Changing myself was not enough: the world, too, would have to change for me to be happy.

Not every Alexander pupil goes through what I did, or goes through it to the degree that I did. I think I was particularly removed from the ideal I have described when I started my lessons, and I have since made this ideal the central goal of my life. Therefore, my voyage has been longer than most, and my goal will remain unreachable by definition. All the same, the changes I went through and the turmoil I experienced as a result are common enough during Alexander lessons. In effect, depending on the pupil's needs and wants, the turmoil that accompanies change is an *inevitable*, *necessary*, and *desirable* effect of a committed study of the Alexander Technique.

PERSONAL RELATIONSHIPS

Turmoil occurs in various guises during Alexander training. Many people have for a long time made professional and personal decisions based not on their true desires and capabilities, but on their *perceived* ones. Because of faulty sensory awareness, a gap exists between perception and reality, between what we do and what we feel we do, between who we are and who we think we are. As this gap narrows – as an Alexander pupil begins to use him or herself better, thereby better gauging both himself or herself and the world around – decisions taken in the past start to appear doubtful or wrong: wrong career, wrong job, wrong lifestyle, wrong marriage.

These new perceptions, which can arrive gradually or suddenly, may be painful and even destructive, although to destroy chains is to free oneself. I believe that the Technique has triggered the end of many relationships. I choose my words carefully: 'triggered', not 'caused'. A partner in an unsatisfactory marriage may acquire, through lessons in the Technique, a better understanding of the causes and symptoms of his or her dissatisfaction. Simple as it is, the framework of the Technique gives clear insights into human nature. An end-gainer is somebody whose sensory awareness is faulty. Alexander pupils who learn to end-gain less in the course of lessons, and who start to perceive others as either end-gainers or non-end-gainers, may find it increasingly harder to live with partners or lovers who habitually end-gain and who inhibit and direct poorly. Indeed, even kissing a badly co-ordinated person (and most end-gainers are badly co-ordinated almost by definition) becomes downright unpleasant.

As in all situations, three choices are open to you: get out of the situation altogether; change the situation; or change yourself. It is often hard to judge which is the best strategy.

Kissing

Kissing presents some interesting kinaesthetic challenges. A tall partner tends to stoop and reach down to the shorter one, misusing himself (or herself) in the process. Unwittingly, the shorter partner aggravates the problem by making herself (or himself) shorter still. Look at how the Egyptian actress Maryam Fakhr ed Dine, in a scene from *Risalat Gharam*, takes her head back and down as she gazes into the eyes of Kamal al Chinnawi. She contracts her head into her neck and rounds her back and shoulders. For a man to kiss a woman whose neck and spine lack tone is startling, even unpleasant, like trying to play a violin with a loosened bow.

Magda, another Egyptian actress, uses herself in a wholly different manner. She lengthens her neck, which becomes a natural extension of her spine, and makes herself taller – and more enticing – even as she tips her head backwards. This makes the act of kissing Farid al Atrache (in a scene from *Min Agl Hobbi*) kinaesthetically easier, and, one imagines readily, more satisfying for both partners.

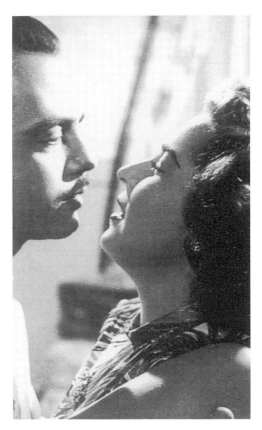 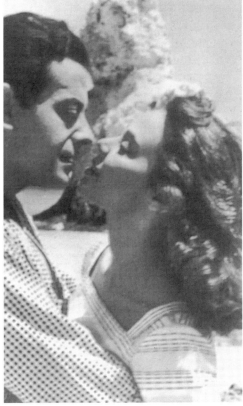

People who work hard at sustaining their marriages are admirable. People who know when and how to quit an unsustainable marriage are admirable too. Nevertheless, the one strategy that is richest in its possibilities is to change yourself, before changing a marriage or giving up on it.

In Chapter 3, I quoted Alexander on the essence of a lesson. His words are pertinent to the subject of personal relationships, and I wish to quote them again: 'You are not here to do exercises,' he said, 'or to learn to do something right, but to get able to meet a stimulus that always puts you wrong and to learn to deal with it.'[18] I often say to my pupils that their reactions in any given situation may be either *normal* (as everybody else's, as they have always been) or *natural* (according to the laws of nature, as they should ideally be). The object of Alexander lessons is to help you change your reactions in all situations from normal to natural. This applies to personal interactions too, intimate or not, in which you meet endless stimuli that put you wrong.

When you first start studying the Alexander Technique, you are likely to want to change the world and make it more Alexander-like. You will have the same impulse regarding the inhabitants of the world, especially those nearest to you. This was certainly my heart's desire after I discovered the Technique, and it resulted in great unhappiness. Later you will see (as I did myself) that the best thing you can do, for yourself and for the world, is to *change yourself*, not the world. The world is not Alexander-like; neither are other people. The only way you can make the world – or others – more Alexander-like is to make yourself be so. People with whom you are intimately involved – parents and siblings, a spouse, a lover, your in-laws – will then have good reasons to thank you for the Technique.

NON-DOING

We have all been in difficult situations which become ever more difficult the harder we try to affect them. As I wrote earlier, the Technique gives you the ability not to react. This is the best response to a large number of situations, as well as a pre-condition to all healthy reaction. Before you can do the right thing, you have to be able to do nothing, the better to lower the probability of doing the wrong thing.

Here is an illustration of this general principle. Your child is crying. Before you can do the right thing (to console her, perhaps) you have to be able to do nothing (and let her express her unhappiness until she runs out of unhappiness), the better to lower the probability of doing the wrong thing (to yell at her or to hit her, which would make her cry harder).

Alexander liked drawing a distinction between something complex and something complicated. A series of essentially simple factors brought together would constitute a complex arrangement, the parts of which remain simple – a composition by J. S. Bach, for instance, or a Swiss watch. Within complication, however, there is nothing simple – as demonstrated by political conflicts such as those in the Balkans or in Ireland. High emotions dictate much of what happens in political life, in which the difference between doing and non-doing may well be the difference between life and death. During a moment of deep crisis in his Middle Eastern country, a journalist wrote in a prestigious daily: 'We don't care any more what they will do, the main thing is to do something.'[19] It is curious to observe how we wish that somebody *else*—the infamous 'they' of this journalist's plea—do something, perhaps in the hope of ridding ourselves from the responsibility for the situation that confronts us. Yet every action undertaken in this spirit ('the main thing is to do something') only renders a complicated situation ever more complicated, and usually at

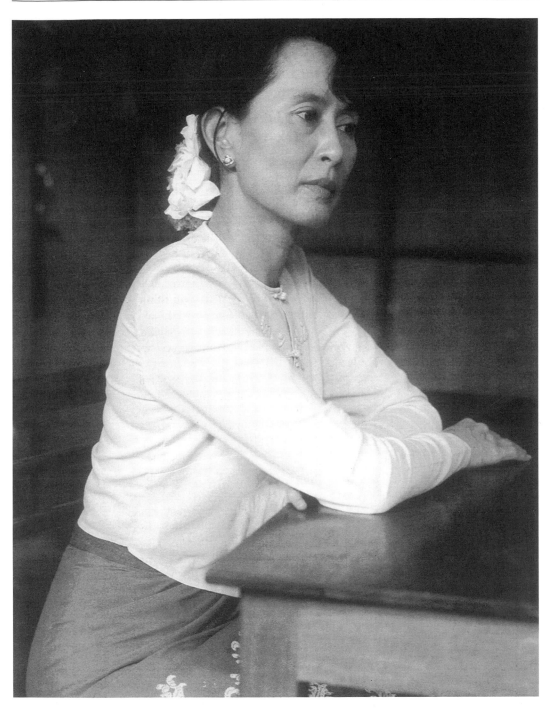

Restraint in the face of brutal provocation. Aung San Suu Kyi, Nobel Peace Prize.

enormous human costs. The journalist above undoubtedly expressed the feelings of many of his fellow countrymen and women. I wonder if they expressed equally unanimous regret when the actions of their government, prodded by public sentiment, sowed destruction all around them.

Another journalist, writing elsewhere about demagoguery, struck a different note: 'When we do not know anymore what to do, we tend to do any old thing. Or to do too much. This we call distress.'[20] If distressed, do not act; first find ways of lessening your distress. Then, and only then, decide on a course of action. Letting things be and leaving others alone is a powerful tool for changing the world. Much of what goes wrong today is the effect of our wilfully trying to control or change what is uncontrollable or unchangeable. Disinterested detachment need not be confused with callous indifference. It is possible to be passionate *and* compassionate without being interfering or domineering. The father who lets his child cry may have as much or more wisdom than the one who tries to comfort her. Obviously, each situation has to be assessed anew and afresh. All the same, once you give up the urge to control situations and people, you may well be surprised to find out how productive doing nothing really is. I like saying that there are many kinds of nothing, and that it is possible to do the right nothing and the wrong nothing. Bad English, perhaps, but a useful reminder that everything depends on circumstance and context, as I argued earlier. Doing nothing, then, is the right thing to do if the situation demands it and if you know how to do nothing.

BEING WRONG

End-gaining affects every area of human endeavour, including politics, science, reli-

gion, arts, sports, and nutrition. Naturally, it affects every area of *your* life, and if you stop end-gaining you will benefit immeasurably. Before things get better, however, they may well get worse. Incipient self-awareness is a state akin to self-consciousness. When you first wake up to the constant manifestations of wrongful end-gaining, you may despair of your every gesture. You sit and stand wrongly, you walk, breathe, and speak wrongly, you work and play and make love and sleep wrongly. The harder you strive for rightness, the deeper you sink into wrongness.

Resourceful pupils will positively enjoy the discovery of their faulty sensory awareness. To feel new sensations, even of wrong things newly detected, is a source of pleasure. Alexander used to say, 'Don't come to me unless, when I tell you you are wrong, you make up your mind to smile and be pleased.'[19] Most people want to *be* right, to *feel* that they are right (not the same thing), and to *be seen to be* right (which does not depend upon being right or feeling right). Nothing, I think, can do more for your own self-esteem than liberating yourself from the fear of being wrong, feeling wrong, or being seen to be wrong.

Indeed, experienced Alexandrians enjoy defusing conflicts by admitting to being wrong, *even when they know for a fact that they are right*. I excuse myself to a stranger who shoves me in the street. He is likely to become civil on the spot – disarmed, as it were. And if he does not, so what? You need not be apathetic and subservient; assume your wrongness, real or pretended, with a proud bearing and a sanguine demeanour. Admitting to being wrong is much more fun than being afraid of being wrong.

Glimpsing an ideal will surely tempt you to attain it, yet to hanker for rightness is to endgain. The Alexander Technique is about a journey, not a destination. It does not matter how far you have gone already, or how far you have to go; all that matters is to be on the right road. Straight is the gate, and narrow is the way. Once you find yourself on this lovely path, you will stop fretting about being right or being wrong, and you may even smile, if only inwardly, when others prove you wrong.

THE TECHNIQUE AND PSYCHOTHERAPIES

In the light of what I have written so far, several questions suggest themselves about the Alexander Technique and human psychology. Are the principles of the Technique compatible with those of psychoanalysis and other forms of therapy? Can the Technique obviate the need for therapy? Inversely, can successful therapy obviate the need for Alexander lessons?

I think that it is almost impossible to consider a set of principles separately from the way these principles are individually practised. The term 'Alexander Technique' encompasses as many different practices as there are different teachers. Even two teachers trained at the same time in the same school will remain distinct in their beliefs, abilities, goals, and methods. This is inevitable and, to a large extent, desirable. It applies equally to psychoanalysis and to all other schools of human thought.

Alexander teacher A works in a manner that is downright contradictory to the practice of psychoanalyst B. Alexander teacher C, however, works in a manner that complements psychoanalyst's D. Are the Technique and psychoanalysis, then, complementary or contradictory? This must be determined on an individual basis, according to the teacher, the analyst, and the pupil or client, as well as time and circumstance.

Many pupils first seek an Alexander teacher for a problem they perceive as physical, and most clients seek therapists for a problem they perceive as mental. I have already argued that

such a separation does not exist, and that lessons in the Alexander Technique affect the whole person. (I expect that analysts and other therapists argue the same for their work.) Even if we accept this as axiomatic, the question remains: Are there mental conditions beyond the reach of the Alexander Technique?

The simple answer is yes, but we must consider many aspects of the question. The late Wilfred Barlow, who was both a medical doctor and a certified Alexander teacher, stated the following in his book *The Alexander Principle*: 'I have never yet seen a neurotic person who did not show dystonic patterns'[20] (in other words, who did not misuse himself). We could argue (with the help of William James) that, to a degree, neurosis *is* misuse. Eliminating misuse often mitigates neurosis, and eliminates it in some cases.

Misuse is equally present in more serious psychological conditions. These too respond to a change in the use of the sufferer, although this change may not be enough in itself. In such cases the Technique can be an extremely useful complement to therapy, without replacing it. Some Alexander pupils who have undergone therapy at the same time as taking lessons have credited the Technique with making their therapies particularly productive.

For many Alexander pupils, things may get worse before they can become better. This is often necessary and inevitable, yet some people are unable to handle the discoveries of 'being wrong'. It may also be that such discoveries are altogether unavailable to some. It seems clear to me that a person going through a psychotic episode needs first and foremost the good care of modern medicine, which produces ever more sophisticated and effective drugs, including those that act upon the mind.

In short, the Alexander Technique may by itself fundamentally alter a psychological condition; it may be an adjunct to therapy; or, in a few instances, it may have potentially

A few years ago, an operation brought an end to years of pain for me. Thanks to the operation, I suddenly felt renewed, and more alive than I had for a long time, yet I imagined that the years of illness had probably affected my posture. I also thought to myself that health must be more than the absence of illness. This led me to look for an Alexander teacher.

I came to Alexander hoping to improve my posture and to lessen the tension in my life. As the lessons unfolded, I was astonished by the accompanying effects on my mental state. External events had long prompted a familiar reflex of anxiety: fear of making mistakes, fear of failure, fear of success, fear of being disliked, fear of being in some way responsible for the 'starving millions', the disappearance of the rain forest, World War III ... As I experienced the release of tension, I let go of all that, and I survived intact!

Instead of reacting with anxiety to the world around me, I now see the endless possibilities for self-realization, for love, for fulfilment. This has been a positive and life-enhancing insight, but also emotionally overwhelming.

I feel empowered at last, totally in charge of myself. As a result of this new-found strength, I can put space between me and a person or situation that seems threatening. My reaction now incorporates a little *moment of choice*, which allows me to decide how to react. I feel anchored to a centre of gravity. Nothing can damage my essential being.

I no longer feel obliged to take on responsibility for others' reactions to me, or for their suffering. I can empathize or sympathize, I can give constructive help, yet I can refuse the agonizing burden of responsibility which often leads to that destructive 'I was only trying to

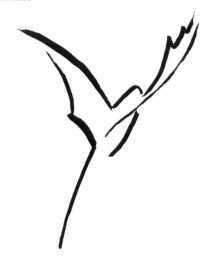

help' approach. My changed awareness of myself seems to produce positive effects on external events around me. I now relate to other people not in terms of the effect they have on me, but in terms of their own attempts to deal with reality as they perceive it. I can see past the surface words or actions, through to the basic elements of humanness we have in common.

I feel suffused with serenity: I find that I am smiling at people in the street for no apparent reason. My thought processes have gained a fluidity and adaptability which enable me to cope easily with change. I feel a wonderful combination of what might be called 'spiritual transcendence' and animal awareness of myself as a biological, harmonious organism. For me now, there is no distinction between 'mind' and 'body': there is only one being, one consciousness, free from any judgement of good and bad, moral and immoral. Life is just 'life'. Good-bye, Descartes – and thank you, F.M. Alexander.

harmful effects. (This does not disprove the Technique in any way; psychosis may be almost intractable in many cases.)

The mechanics of psychological change in Alexander lessons differ from those of therapy. Teachers often receive intimate confidences from their pupils, but such exchanges are not essential for a pupil to learn how to inhibit and direct. Indeed, unless an Alexander teacher has received additional training as a therapist, he or she should either gently discourage these confidences or listen to them without reacting. A teacher cannot be all things to all pupils; a good teacher avoids becoming a parent figure, confessor or therapist.

Psychologically, the work of the Alexander Technique is perhaps more related to Zen Buddhism and the teaching of Krishnamurti: changes happen not in connection with a dissection of childhood dreams, familial relationships, or sexuality, but more as a result of an insight in the here and now. Your old self did not 'think up', and its personality was largely determined by this fact. Right now you are 'thinking up', and this determines whom you have become.

A pupil who was often depressed complained to me once that, although she felt marvellous walking out of her lessons, she fell back into depression sooner or later. It may take a long time to make psychological changes permanent, but this does not change the fact that the Alexander Technique causes profound changes – proof of that is that my pupil was transformed at the end of every lesson. No serious psychotherapist would promise quick and permanent changes; Alexander teachers can promise no more.

If the Technique can, in some cases, lessen or eliminate the need for therapy, can therapy also make Alexander lessons unnecessary? I described an Alexander lesson in Chapter 4. I argued that, since mind and body are one, it should be possible to move towards the Alexandrian ideal without experiencing the touch of an Alexander teacher, but through a change in mental habits and conceptions instead. This is possible, but only *with great difficulty*, due to the vicious circle of faulty sensory awareness and misuse of the self. 'Insights which you may get when in a very disturbed state of USE are not necessarily to be trusted,'[21] Dr Barlow wrote. This is not to dismiss psychotherapy, which has paid great service to many people, but to point out the limits that it may have in certain situations; naturally, this is also the case with the Alexander Technique.

To summarize a discussion with many facets, the aims and methods of the Alexander Technique, as practised by many (but not all) teachers, may be removed from those of psychoanalysis and other forms of psychotherapy, as practised by many (but not all) therapists. Psychotherapy and the Alexander Technique have different limits, and play rôles that may be complementary, overlapping, or contradictory to each other, depending on the particular situation.

For some observers, the Alexander Technique has seemed akin to classical conditioning, and perhaps to behavioural therapy. Yet, as I pointed out when discussing inhibition and direction, the Technique differs fundamentally from classical conditioning. The dog of the Pavlovian cliché salivates upon hearing the bell. An Alexandrian dog, if it existed, would hear the bell, not react at first, and then choose a course of action or inaction as the case may be.

H.W. Fowler, the lexicographer, discussed the difference between instinct and intuition briefly in his *Modern English Usage*: 'While both, as faculties, are contrasted with that of reason, intuition is the attribute by which gods and angels, saints and geniuses, are superior to the need of reasoning, and instinct is the gift by which animals are compensated for their inability to reason.' Quoting the English essayist and poet Joseph Addison, Fowler concluded that 'our Superiors are guided by intuition, and our Inferiors by instinct'.[22]

I believe that the Alexander Technique, if not making us more like gods and angels, certainly lifts us from the condition of animals salivating at the sound of a bell. Alexander called the ability to inhibit 'Man's Supreme Inheritance' (the title of the first of his four books). To inhibit is to decide, *for yourself*, how best to react in any given situation, and to have the ability to carry out your own decisions. There could be no greater source of individual empowerment and emotional well-being.

CHAPTER 6
Health and Well-Being

I HAVE LIVED THROUGH IT – EDWARD, 32, WRITER AND BROKER

It is four o'clock in the morning. I wake up with a chill, lying on my side, uncovered, naked. The nurses are about to spin me for the third time in six hours. The spin keeps bedridden patients from developing bedsores and body bruises. Two nurses position themselves on either side of the bed, grab the sheets on which I lie, then lift and pull me across to the very edge of the bed – the abyss – while they bend me into the foetal position. My chest leaning against her, the first nurse jerks the sheets upwards on her side of the bed and spins me backwards towards the second nurse. For what seems an eternity, all of my weight rests on the hole in my back, from which the surgeon plucked my herniated disc ten days earlier. The pain is staggering, and I scream as the second nurse halts my collapse on to the floor by lifting the sheets quickly and abruptly on her side. The first nurse covers me, and I breathe a sigh of relief. I try to get two hours' sleep before they come back to start all over again – twelve times a day for two weeks.

Genesis of a Problem

This is a cautionary tale of end-gaining and misuse, a story of interest to anybody who is curious about the Alexander Technique. As a child I was badly co-ordinated, overweight, and unfit. I lacked confidence on the playing field and fumbled things when under pressure. I can see now that this early lack of co-ordination and the embarrassment it caused me were at the heart of my drive later in life to excel at any cost in all things physical.

I had the first of many injuries aged twelve, playing American football. When I breathed in deeply or turned my torso, I felt like someone had stuck a knife in between my shoulder blades and was twisting it. The custom at the time (as it is today in many circles) was to train through the pain. I simply continued to play the game, and the pain eventually went away.

I remember my mother, a long-suffering victim of sciatica, admonishing me to lift with my knees, not with my back, as I worked around the house. The advice was good, but not the model: she herself often lifted heavy objects with her lower back and arms, as did everybody else around me. I ignored the advice and imitated the model, and continued to lift and shift heavy objects with no regard for the well-being of my back.

Throughout my adolescence, I attempted to keep up with older men who were bigger, stronger, and more experienced than me – working at a construction site when I was thirteen, for example. As a lifeguard on the beach, I tried to impress young women by doing, on my own, the heavy work that was normally done by three men.

I was an overweight and over-active adolescent. From the age of fifteen onwards, the strain of girth on my lower back caused constant pain, relieved only when I was able to get my weight down and my stomach into shape to support my spine. I tried to ease my pain by following a harsh regimen of stretches. I did not know that the stretching put yet more pressure on the discs. The discs were irritating the nerves, which sent signals to my brain to freeze the muscles and protect the spinal cord from further damage. I felt the frozen muscles, but totally misread the signal. I thought the tight muscles simply needed more stretching, and continued to exercise, ignoring the complaints of my body.

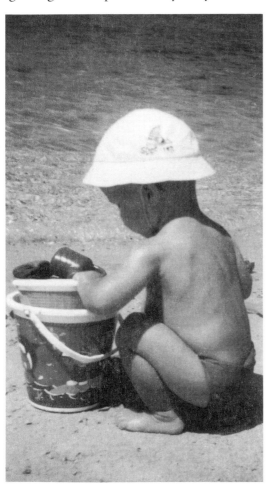

The Onset of Crisis

In my early twenties I was introduced to circus skills and became active in theatre. I learned to juggle with balls, clubs, torches, knives, tennis rackets, and anything else that came to hand. I learned to ride a unicycle, walk on a slack rope, run on stilts, and swallow flaming torches. I discovered that if I worked at something for long enough, my muscles would eventually find the rhythm of the activity. I got the results I was after, but the constant repetition and the excessive tension were storing up problems for later on.

Within a year of learning these skills I began to make a living on stage, and pushed myself constantly in performance. Sometimes this was necessary, because executing certain routines incorrectly could be dangerous or life-threatening. It hurts to fall off a five-foot unicycle or to catch the wrong end of a burning torch. Paradoxically, by not making mistakes in my tricks I made unreasonable demands on my body – a mistake greater than the ones I was trying to avoid. I became extremely fit, yet incredibly tense in my back and shoulders. I even managed to pull a muscle in my neck while putting in a contact lens. Clearly, something had to change.

Over the years I tried to solve my back problems with a variety of practices, including yoga – which I found difficult to incorporate into my daily life – and massage and chiropractic, which helped for brief periods without addressing the root of the problem.

Some eight years ago, a friend offered me a book about the Alexander Technique. I was impressed by the simple logic of what I read that the way one uses something determines its functioning, both current and future. Suffering from so much pain, I was open to learning how to use myself better in the hope of reducing it. I took a few lessons after reading the book, but had to interrupt them to go on tour with my show. On the plane out to Japan my lower back was hurting, and, for the first time, my left leg as well. I attributed the pain to sitting for too long in a crowded plane. I had a hectic time on arrival, only going to bed a jet-lagged wreck many hours later. In the middle of my first performance the following day, I felt a sharp click in my back. I finished the show, and afterwards I felt pins and needles in both legs. I tried to mitigate my discomfort with hot packs, hot baths, massage, and stretching. Although the symptoms did not disappear, I was able to finish the tour. Back in Paris, I saw several specialists, including a neurosurgeon, a chiropractor, and a physiotherapist.

The advice I received included things like drinking more water to inflate the discs, keeping my back warm, cooling it, and having it manipulated. I can see now that the best advice I got was to do nothing: take a break, lie down, and let my back heal itself. However, I had another contract in Japan, and soon I was back on stage. Through a combination of gentle warming up, rest, and massage, I managed to get through the tour without further injury, although I was still plagued by lower back pain and the pins and needles in my legs.

Back in Paris, the difficulty in using my left leg became ever greater. Finally, after a fall during an improvisation, the back of my leg was paralysed completely from the buttocks down. I consulted the neurologist again, who became quite agitated and did his best to get me an appointment that same afternoon with a surgeon at a large Paris hospital. The surgeon soon suggested I go straight upstairs and get prepared for an operation the following morning on my spine. He explained that the operation would free my spinal nerves quickly, and perhaps restore my leg to near its previous strength. Without the operation I would walk with a limp for the rest of my life, and might even lose control of my bladder and sexual function.

I was traumatized by what he told me, and decided to seek second, third, and fourth opinions in the course of the next 24 hours. Everyone I consulted was perfectly clear: I had to have the operation or I would limp for life. Nerves are damaged under excessive pressure, and the only hope for partial recovery was to get the pressure off my nerves as soon as possible by surgically removing the disc and getting impulses from the brain moving through the area again.

After the operation I spent two weeks in hospital suffering the painful indignities described earlier. The operation is quite common for people who have misused themselves for sixty years, but it takes a special effort to achieve the same wear and tear by my age – I was twenty-five at the time. Even more than the pain and paralysis I had suffered in the years before the operation, my experience of the hospital was instrumental in focusing my energies on improving my use, so I would never have to go back there again.

Unfortunately, I had not quite learnt my lesson yet. Combining enthusiasm and stupidity, I exerted myself recklessly after my operation and ended up prolonging my recovery by several months. After six months – the recovery time predicted by my doctors – I was not even able to sit down for more than fifteen minutes, much less perform on stage.

New Discoveries

When my savings ran out I had to take a job that was physically less demanding than street theatre. Changing careers left me unhappy, but provided me with a steady income and allowed me to pay for regular Alexander lessons. I learned quickly that I was far more messed up than I realized. I looked muscular and fit, yet I was carrying loads of tension, stiffness, and injury, which I had been ignoring for too long. I had misused myself for years before being crippled by pain; I now understood that it would take more than a few lessons to unlearn the habits that had got me there in the first place.

If you do something wrong for long enough, it begins to feel right. What is right then feels wrong. In one of my early lessons my teacher put me into a position in which I felt like I was balancing on my toes, with my left shoulder leaning forwards and my chest pushed backwards. After the lesson, however, many of my aches and pains began to melt away, and I realized that the new position was indeed a better way to stand, my initial discomfort notwithstanding. I discovered that the origin of pain was rarely in the place where I felt the pain itself. I realized that my headaches were caused by tension in my neck. I thought the tension in my neck was caused by chronic tension in my shoulder, but found that the problem in my shoulder was the result of compensating for a vertebra in my dorsal spine that was out of place. I had not noticed that the vertebra was out of place until I started to breathe fully again, which caused pain in the ribs that had been frozen for such a long time. It took several years of lessons for me to understand that much of my pain was caused by an injury to the middle of my back that I could not even feel when I started lessons – possibly the original injury I had suffered while playing football in my youth. I know now that I constructed a pattern of misuse around the injury, compensating for it and masking the pain (by freezing my left shoulder in an unnatural position, for instance), but creating new problems elsewhere. As I stopped compensating, I sometimes felt new pains, yet these seemed healthy: they were the pains of moving normally again after being long stuck in the wrong position.

For a long time I alternated between feeling good in lessons and hurting from craning my neck forward and upward, trying too hard to force a process that is about not forcing anything. My whole life had been one of achieving results through physical or mental strength, and the end-gainer in me found 'unlearning' difficult. I would have given up had it not been for the sheer physical joy that I experienced in the lessons themselves, which I could occasionally reproduce at home, when I lay on my back and simply gave myself directions.

Practical Results

Learning the Technique may be slow and frustrating, but it has many benefits. The most noticeable to my friends and family was improved posture and increased height. For a year after I started my lessons, old friends kept on remarking that I had grown since we last met. I am not sure if my height had really increased, or whether I simply looked taller because I was carrying myself differently.

I have enjoyed remarkable health through the last six years, and have missed only four days of work due to ill health. By directing my use I tap into my body's capacity to regenerate itself. Today I can choose whether to have pain or not. I can decide to continue misusing myself (and suffer pain as the price of my misuse), or to slow down, inhibit, and direct my use (thereby reducing or eliminating pain).

My most recent success with the Technique was on a skiing holiday. I had not been on skis for ten years, and I was nervous about the possibility of re-injuring my back. Despite my trepidation, I found that, by directing my head forward and up and my back back and up, I was able to ski more easily than I remembered in my youth. I felt as if I was up away from the mountain, instead of down into it. My speed was unchanged, yet inside my mind I seemed to be going more slowly. I was therefore better able to spot and deal with the changing terrain as it rushed up to meet me, and with other skiers as they came into my field of vision. Although I was much less fit than I had been on my ski trip ten years earlier, the experience of skiing changed from an arduous fight against my skis and the mountain to a fluid and relaxed descent.

I have learned from the Technique that sometimes I must slow down to run faster, and I take fifteen minutes each day at lunch to lie down and direct myself – a better use of time than taking coffee breaks or having long lunches. I do not sleep in these moments of constructive rest, and find that they leave me refreshed and ready for business in a way that coffee and adrenalin, my old standbys, never did. I work as a commodities broker, and the stress of the marketplace and of constant phone calls is not always compatible with good use. Even when I misuse myself at work, however, I now have the tools to restore my body quickly to a balanced resting state.

In an apparent paradox, as I have done less I have earned more. I have gradually stopped doing things at the last minute, because I am unwilling to misuse myself to finish a project or make a deadline. Now I inhibit myself from using the precious resources at my disposal on tasks that are unimportant. I receive fewer accolades for superhuman achievements, but those achievements had always been the result of costly end-gaining. Today my goal is not to achieve more than others, but simply to use myself well while living a full and balanced life, active yet serene.

Emotionally, I found that my need to force things to change has gone. Rather than worrying about what happens 'to me' in my life, I am better able to deal with difficulties as they present themselves – often by relaxing instead of tensing up. Inhibiting the 'fight or flight' reflexes allows for a considered response to most situations. To stay 'up and back' in crisis might also just be called 'keeping your head.'

The Technique has made my body a much more comfortable place to live. It has given me the joyous experience of breathing freely and just *being*. I was looking only for a solution to a physical problem – which I found – but I have been given tools to develop the mental and spiritual dimensions of my life as well. For that, I am profoundly grateful.

PAIN IS A GREAT TEACHER

Every life is unique, including Edward's. He has lived through a set of events that nobody else in this world has ever encountered. The people he has met and the sensations and feelings he has experienced are all exclusively his. His life is therefore original and extraordinary, as are yours and mine, yet his experiences have a certain universal resonance as well. His background, the nature of his problems, and the difficulties he faced in solving them are all similar to those of many other people who have sought out the help of an Alexander teacher. Behind each of Edward's experiences lies a general principle that manifests itself in the lives of thousands of men and women. His testimonial is an invaluable study in the applications of the Technique to health and well-being.

Each Alexander pupil has his or her own specific reason for taking Alexander lessons. Nevertheless, the majority of pupils start their lessons because of pain, which they themselves characterize as 'physical', be it skeletal or muscular. The pain may be due to tendonitis, arthritis, osteoporosis, Repetitive Strain Injury, the after-effects of an operation, an accident, a birth defect, or a dozen other causes. In Edward's case, the immediate cause of his pain was a slipped disc in his spine.

We often hear it said that 'pain is a great teacher'. Pain is an obvious incentive for self-examination, change, and growth. This is not to say that you need to be suffering from pain to take Alexander lessons. Many pupils come for their first lessons completely free from any pain, and benefit greatly all the same. Indeed, ideally, a pupil should come to the Technique before he or she starts suffering from the effects of end-gaining and misuse, and apply the Technique for prevention rather than cure. Edward end-gained for too long, and the misuse caused by his end-gaining finally caught up with him. Had he learned in his youth about end-gaining and misuse, as well as inhibition and direction, he might have saved himself all the pain and humiliation that he describes in his testimonial.

I write of 'prevention' and 'cure' advisedly. The Technique is not a strictly therapeutic method. Rather, it is pedagogical in nature, and the relation between an Alexander teacher and his or her pupil is not the same as that between therapist and client. I cannot 'cure' Edward. I can only help him become better aware of his habits of use and teach him ways of changing them, or, better still, teach him to stop doing the wrong thing. If he really stops doing the wrong thing, he will first stop damaging himself, and then allow his organism to regenerate itself. I can teach him to stop end-gaining, but I cannot cure him.

THE CAR AND THE DRIVER

Consciously or not, we tend to think of our bodies as mechanical in nature, and our physical problems as similar to those of a car that has broken down. This may be a useful analogy, as long as we realize that the problem is not that our 'car' has defective parts, but rather that we are terrible drivers. We need therefore to go back to driving school, instead of taking the car to the mechanic.

Edward's problems came about because he end-gained in everything that he did – in

sports, working around the house, in his first jobs in adolescence, and as a clown and acrobat. By end-gaining, he misused himself. The misuse strained his body, and the strain resulted in pain. It would be difficult, if not impossible, for him to free himself permanently from pain without eliminating his habit of end-gaining. Since he end-gained in all that he did, he had to change his whole life in order to get rid of the pain.

A few observations suggest themselves. First, when end-gaining is the ultimate cause of pain, methods of mechanical manipulation may mitigate or eliminate it in the short term, without freeing the sufferer from it. Edward's experiences with massage and chiropractic demonstrate the point. These and other methods, such as osteopathy, may indeed offer relief from pain, but they are unlikely to eliminate its cause – the universal habit of end-gaining.

Permanent change comes only when you stop doing the wrong thing. In some cases, manipulative methods have worsened a condition or reinforced a person's tendency to do the wrong thing. Repeated clicking of joints, for instance, may weaken them in the long term. If Alexander's concept of non-doing makes sense to you (as I hope it does at this point in the book), you would do well to approach all manipulative practices with circumspection. However, it is also true that a sensitive, well-trained, and experienced massage practitioner or osteopath may offer very effective short-term solutions to tension and pain; in some cases, practitioners of these methods know of better short-term solutions than those in the repertory of an Alexander teacher. To return to the analogy about the car and its driver, it is possible to solve some problems with a trip to the mechanic, although much less often than we like to believe.

Secondly, the relationship between end-gaining and misuse, and between use and functioning, demonstrates yet again the most important principle of the Alexander Technique: body and mind are inseparable, and our problems cannot be classified as purely 'physical' or purely 'mental'. Comparing the body to a car is in fact false because in reality there exists no distinction whatsoever between the car and the driver, that is, between the thing controlled and the control itself.

This is both good and bad. It is good because to be whole is the finest human attribute. It is bad because many of our difficulties do not have easy solutions; seemingly localized problems, such as tendonitis of the wrist, for example, need to be considered in a context of end-gaining and misuse of the whole self. It is good too because, if you find the right solution to one of your problems, you will solve many other problems in one go, indirectly and automatically. Among such problems, some will seem to you at first to lie beyond the scope of the Alexander Technique; you may well be unaware of others until they are solved.

Edward's main reason for seeking out the Alexander Technique was back pain. Indeed, when he booked his first lesson, I am sure he believed it was the *only* reason for him to see an Alexander teacher. However, his pain was just a symptom of a condition that permeated his whole being. In the absence of a Greek or Latin name for it, let us call this condition 'end-gaining and misuse'! In his testimonial, Edward tells us how he found out quickly that he was much more messed up than he thought. Changing his condition took time, effort, money, perseverance, patience, and even a little faith. In the end, though, he got rid of his initial complaint and benefited in many different ways – emotional, intellectual, personal, and professional.

The human body is not really an arrangement of more or less rigid parts joined together with a series of hinges and articulations, like a car or a machine. Neither is it a pile of blocks or bricks, like a house, which needs to be aligned in a symmetrical balance. The living body, the body that laughs and cries, the body that ails and heals, is a complex system of energies that flow along curved paths; these paths cannot always be measured or even visualized. The natural curves of the human body and the curved paths along which energies flow make it particularly tricky for you to try to sit or stand 'straight'. You are better off 'thinking up along the spine', a dynamic formulation which lessens the danger of your holding yourself in rigid positions.

Beautiful as they may be, cars, machines, and houses are static and inorganic, and relatively easy to dissect, analyse, operate, and fix. Human beings are lively, ever-changing, unpredictable, subject to instinct, intuition, imagination, humour and passion, and, in the end, impossible to understand and control. If you need an analogy, abandon the image of a car in favour of that of a river or a whole ecosystem, where myriad forms of life coexist in interdependence – sometimes successfully, sometimes disastrously, always imponderably.

COMPENSATING MECHANISMS

Edward speaks of creating layers of tension to 'protect' his shoulder. Thanks to this compensating mechanism, his shoulder hurts less for a while. Yet, in the long run, all compensating mechanisms lead to a deterioration in the use of the self and, consequently, in functioning. This may affect both the body part meant to be protected and the rest of the body as well.

You may have had the experience, for example, of walking with blisters on your foot. In order to lessen the discomfort in your foot, you walk with a limp, hesitantly, trying not to put weight on the blisters. Before long your hips hurt, and then your spine and your neck. You are paying too high a price for your compensating mechanisms.

Because of faulty sensory awareness, it is possible not to be conscious of the compensating mechanism, or even of the problem the mechanism is supposed to help. Edward talks of spending years unaware of an old injury to his middle back. As he attempted, unconsciously, to protect this injury, he created a whole chain of tensions that affected his neck and shoulders, his vertebrae and his breathing, resulting in discomfort, pain, and headaches.

The Alexander Technique helps you to become aware of the existence of a problem, its manifestations, its consequences, and its effects throughout the organism. The problem may be an old injury, its manifestation pain, its consequence a compensating mechanism, and its effects the misuse and tension of body parts far removed from the original injury.

Compensating mechanisms that create excessive tension and misuse are by definition negative. There are, however, equally positive compensating mechanisms. To use yourself well means to use your back and legs quite actively; the better you use your back and legs, the freer your neck and shoulders become. In the event of an injury or illness, using your back and legs more actively than you do habitually may improve the functioning of the whole organism so much that the injury heals more easily. Indeed, the best way of inhibiting negative compensating mechanisms is to activate positive ones. Edward firmed up his spine and started using his legs in a vigorous and balanced manner, to support his whole upper body. He was therefore able to release his neck and shoulders – which till then had tended to over-work because of lazy legs – thereby freeing his breathing.

Note that this was not a wholly comfortable process. Edward remarks that he experienced new pains as he released old tensions. It is common for an Alexander pupil to encounter bizarre experiences and disagreeable feelings during lessons. All change, however beneficial, causes discomfort. The substance abuser goes through withdrawal symptoms while detoxifying. When a deep cut starts to heal, it itches unbearably. When a professional pianist decides to change her technique, her ability to play with fluency decreases before she masters her new technique. Once mastered, though, the new technique proves superior to the old one, and the discomfort of losing fluency for a while will then seem like a reasonable price to pay for greater mastery.

TO DO, OR NOT TO DO

Edward relates that, as a child, he was badly co-ordinated and unfit, which motivated him later in life to excel in every physical activity. In his attempts to solve what he saw as a problem (his lack of co-ordination), he gave himself a bigger problem (the injuries and pain from his end-gaining and misuse).

This is again a specific manifestation of a universal tendency: that is to fight wrong with wrong (often, but not always, fighting a wrong with its contrary). We do this in every type of activity, in daily life, in personal relationships, in politics and economics. It is such a prevalent habit that we tend to think it is 'natural' to do it. Consider, for example, Edward's regimen of stretches, which he followed in the hope of lessening the tension in his body. By his own admission, the stretches put even more pressure on his discs and nerves, aggravating the situation rather than helping it. Yet there are always experts who advise such stretches, and listeners who heed their advice because they feel that they must *do something*.

Two wrongs do not make a right. If you do something wrong, the only logical course of action is to stop doing it. Doing nothing is often the only thing that you have to do to solve a problem. In many other instances, doing nothing is an essential first step in finding the solution to a problem. As Edward remarks, perhaps the best advice that he received about his back was to do nothing, to rest and wait. Many illnesses are self-regulating and self-terminating. Animals in the wild who are injured manage to heal in the total absence of veterinary care, by resting and fasting. Human beings have the same capacity for self-regeneration. Taking a placebo often mitigates the effects of illness, and even cures it in some cases. The placebo triggers a self-healing process. Men and women who are alert, self-aware, and in control of their own reactions may dispense with placebos altogether and trigger the process by inhibiting, directing, and using themselves well.

Non-doing is one of the great difficulties of the Alexander Technique. We are so used to doing something, and to being seen to be doing something, that the very idea of doing nothing seems wrong. As Edward observes, the end-gainer finds it difficult to 'unlearn'. No serious Alexander teacher would claim that it is easy to unlearn how 'to do' and learn how 'not to do'. Still, the rewards of Alexandrian inhibition are so great that they will justify the pupil's best efforts.

NUTRITION AND DIGESTION

Edward mentions in passing a certain change in his daily life, stating in the end of his testimonial that the constructive rest he now takes in his office gives him more energy than his old companion, coffee. This is a glimpse into the relationship between the Alexander Technique and lifestyle habits. I shall come back to the subject of coffee, but for the moment I wish to address one of the most important aspects of daily living: nutrition and digestion.

There is an intimate connection between the way you use yourself and the functioning of your digestive system. A teacher of the Alexander Technique once swallowed a dose of barium and placed himself under the scrutiny of X-rays. He then demonstrated that his digestion slowed down when he misused himself and sped up when he 'thought up along the spine'.

In truth, the effect of the use of the self on digestion, as well as on other functions of the organism, is much more complex and far-reaching than this somewhat crude experiment would lead us to believe. It is astonishing to hear the sounds that come out of a pupil's abdomen as his or her use starts to change during an Alexander lesson. As the pupil lengthens and widens, as some parts of the body are relaxed and the tonus of some other parts is increased, the whole body changes in shape, dimension, and tone. All the organs inside the body now must shift and find their new place in this transformed space. As they move and relax, the organs let their secretions flow more freely and efficiently, and this flow has a song of its own. 'Early on in my lessons,' writes Liz, a 42-year old woman, 'I was aware of a massive release of tension in the abdominal area, as if my intestines were heaving a sigh of relief. Within the first few weeks, I discovered that my bowel movements were easier and more regular than they had ever been: something that years of attempts with laxatives, exercise, and dietary fibre had never been able to accomplish.'

All pupils, men and women, make their own abdominal music, as individual as the timbre of their own voice. Sometimes a pupil is embarrassed by the sounds produced while lying on the teacher's table, but these sounds signal a deep and healthy change, and a movement towards freedom and well-being. (Incidentally, these sounds are more frequent, varied, and noticeable in women than in men, possibly because their reproductive organs are quite sensitive to changes in use. The Technique, used for a long time in pregnancy and childbirth, can undoubtedly be a complementary tool in treating certain gynaecological problems. One of my pupils, who came to the Technique because of a dropping womb, found that the problem disappeared after a series of lessons; in keeping with the logic of the Technique, the dropped womb was not addressed directly at all.)

Alexander claimed that, if you use yourself well, you can be omnivorous without trouble, since both digestion and evacuation are functions of the way you use yourself. It is true that a person's good use (and consequent good functioning) gives him or her a certain freedom not to worry unduly about nutrition and digestion, while somebody whose digestion is made more difficult by misuse has a smaller margin for carelessness and excess. Nevertheless, it does not seem desirable for anyone to be entirely omnivorous. Despite his excellent use, Alexander, who loved food and drink, suffered all his life from a weakness in the lining of his stomach. In my opinion, he would have benefited from a diet somewhat more restricted than the one in which he indulged.

In fact, good use of the self has a double effect. On the one hand, good health (the natural consequence of using yourself well) allows you some leeway in matters of nutrition. On the other hand, a sharpened sensorial perception (also a natural consequence of using yourself well) leads you to avoid foods and beverages that you come to feel are harmful to your health.

Because I use myself well, I realize that alcoholic drinks (which depress the nervous system) quickly make me tired and unenergized, and that a pizza (which is difficult to digest) makes me heavy. Thanks to the Alexander Technique, I now prefer to stay light, alert and energized, and I avoid eating pizzas and drinking alcohol. I have become more resistant to the harmful effects of various stimuli and substances, but at the same time I avoid all that is detrimental to my health, to my well-being, and to my state from moment to moment.

ALEXANDRIAN INHIBITION AND LIFESTYLE

Everyone who wishes to change his or her lifestyle must face the habits of a whole life. After reading my views on alcoholic drinks, you might imagine that I had to summon up a considerable effort of my conscious will to stop drinking. Perhaps you find it discouraging to think that you, too, will need to fight hard to give up a 'bad' habit – smoking, for example, or consuming too much sugar. However, the Technique will have a double effect on your conscious will, which should help you change your habits more easily.

First, when you develop the faculty of inhibition – the capacity not to react automatically and habitually to a stimulus – you become better able to make a decision and to carry it out. Let us imagine that you have a certain health problem that leads you to decide not to smoke a cigarette, not to drink a beer, not to have a dessert; Alexandrian inhibition would make it easier for you to stick to your decision and not to satisfy an impulse or desire.

Second, and rather more importantly, the Alexander Technique causes a change in your impulses and desires themselves, some of which may well disappear. In such a case, it is not necessary any more for you to exert your conscious will not to satisfy a desire, because the desire is simply not there. It costs me absolutely nothing not to drink, since I have no desire to drink whatsoever. (Chocolate, however, is another matter. I find it rather an enjoyable stimulant, and I can quickly become addicted to it.) True inhibition, in Alexander's understanding of the word, does not mean preventing yourself forcefully from drinking or from smoking, but freeing yourself from the wish to drink or smoke. My sobriety is not therefore the sign of a strong will that dominates an impulse; it signals instead the absence of such an impulse.

It goes without saying that the decision to do or not to do something, when based on the effects that such a thing may have on your well-being, does not imply a value judgement on the thing in question. I abstain from drink not because I feel drinking is immoral, but because I like to be sober, and because I simply do not wish to drink. While the Alexander Technique develops your self-restraint, it does not moralize or advocate asceticism. (Ah! Chocolate …)

WEIGHT LOSS

Since it affects desires and impulses, as well as the habits of a lifetime and the workings of the conscious will, the Alexander Technique can be useful for anybody who wishes to lose weight. Weight problems are quite complex, as they include so many interdependent aspects, including psychological, physiological, genetic, cultural, among others. Medically obese men and women who wish to apply the Technique to losing weight would still have to consult an endocrinologist, a psychologist, a nutritionist, or an expert in exercise (depending on their individual needs).

If you follow a diet with a main goal of losing weight, you risk achieving your goal at too high a price. The means determine the ends directly, and the ends determine the means indirectly. It should follow that every intelligent and efficient search for a goal must be centred on the means used, not on the goal. Eating in a manner that is healthy and balanced

has the side effect of helping obese people normalize their weight. (If truly balanced, the ideal diet also leads underweight people to gain weight.) Weight-loss diets, however, may be harmful to your health; therefore, have the courage, perseverance, and wisdom not to follow a weight-loss diet, even if its short-term effects are to your liking; follow instead a healthy and balanced diet, the long-term effects of which will certainly be to help you arrive at your ideal weight.

Your response to my views on weight loss may be that they represent nothing new. Still, it is helpful sometimes to look at an old idea in a new light. The framework of the Alexander Technique would lead you to realize that you end-gain when you follow a weight-loss diet, and that you are better off inhibiting your desire to achieve quick but costly results.

Alexandrian inhibition allows you to change the speed of some of your reactions and habits of daily life. This is not to say that all your reactions should become slower. On the contrary; the person who inhibits well can react quickly, slowly, or not at all, according to the needs of each situation. Yet one of the effects of inhibition is to help someone who tends to eat too quickly to slow down and take more time to chew, which inevitably changes digestion (which, as we all know, starts by the action of saliva in the mouth). In fact, it may well be that somebody eats too much to compensate for inadequate digestion; in such a case, the improvement in digestion that comes from eating more slowly would lead to a decrease in food intake.

Let us consider what Edward said about coffee. His need for a stimulant has decreased thanks to the greater energy he now has, as he uses himself well and rests constructively. If you too use yourself well, you may find yourself free from the need for sources of quick energy such as coffee, tea, and sugary foods; in turn, this should help you lose weight.

We can now draw a general principle of the Alexander Technique from the preceding observations. The Technique affects all aspects of your life, sometimes directly, sometimes indirectly, sometimes both. This is the case with your voice, your posture, the way you relate to other people, and many other aspects of your life, including your habits of eating and drinking. Here is an example of a direct effect of the Alexander Technique: you become better able not to eat a dessert, thanks to the elevating effect of inhibition on your conscious will. Here is an indirect effect: you have less need for the quick bursts of energy that you once gained from desserts, now that you use yourself well and have a constant source of energy. Note that indirect changes are often more profound and more durable than direct ones.

IMPROVING POSTURE

Chapter 2 dealt at length with 'posture', a term often associated with the Alexander Technique. Posture is a useful concept as long as we define it correctly, without separating it from attitude or from movement. Edward remarks that one of the more noticeable effects of the Technique was the improvement in his posture and the increase in his height. Better posture is in fact the visual manifestation of an inner transformation. As Edward says, using yourself better may not necessarily cause an increase in your height and width, but you may well give the impression to others of having grown. Measurable physical changes may take place too. A pupil's body becomes longer and wider, the shoulders spread sideways and apart, the musculature of the back and legs firms up, and the stomach and buttocks take on a different tone.

Try the following experiment. Stand in front of a mirror, looking at yourself in profile.

Crane your head and neck forward, round your upper back, and let your pelvis slide forwards. Your posture then becomes 'abnormal', and you will be able to see the results for yourself, in particular in your stomach area, which is now big and floppy. Go back to your habitual posture, and watch the changes in your physical appearance when you go from an 'abnormal' posture to a 'normal' one. You may now imagine that there would also be an improvement in your physical appearance when you pass form a 'normal' posture to an 'ideal' one. The difficulty of this change is that it entails not your doing the right thing, but

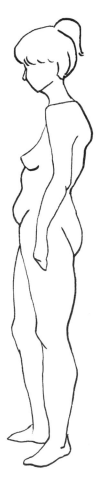

stopping doing the wrong one. Alexander warned his beginner students not to buy new clothes for a while, since the changes in their posture as they learned the Technique were such that soon their dresses or suits would not fit any longer.

I have one last observation to make about excess weight. Everyone who is too heavy should, of course, lose weight, yet it is sometimes exceedingly hard, for all sorts of reasons, for someone to shed enough pounds to approach his or her ideal weight. Ultimately, the overweight person who stays overweight may well learn how to use the Alexander

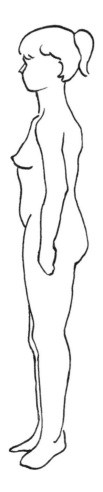

Technique to mitigate the effects of obesity on his or her health. If you learn how to direct your use, you will then move more nimbly and lightly, regardless of weight or bulk, lessening the strain on your skeletal and muscular systems. Remember that there are also trim and fit people whose use is such that they are rather clumsy in their movements. According to the Alexander Technique, such people are 'heavier' than obese men and women who use themselves well.

PREGNANCY AND CHILDBIRTH – CATHERINE DE CHEVILLY

The onset of motherhood is a time when the Alexander Technique proves to be remarkably useful and effective. Since I finished my training as an Alexander teacher in 1991, I have been pregnant twice. Both pregnancies unfolded without complications or difficulties. I was free from back pain throughout, and I gave birth at home with the help of a midwife.

When a woman expects a child, does she really imagine she will go through so many states in such a short time? More than ever, I found it beneficial during my pregnancy to cultivate a certain neutrality, a certain abandon. Such an attitude is contained in the directions: 'I let my neck be free, to let my head go forward and up, to let my back lengthen and widen.' For the being who grows inside of me, for these emotions and feelings, I am just a channel. This thought allows me to create space inside my belly, particularly backwards toward my spinal column, which helps me avoid the typical posture of the pregnant woman – pelvis thrust forwards, lower back hollowed, curves of the spine exaggerated. I create space in my mind, for during pregnancy many memories come to the surface and it is time to allow old wounds to be healed. I create space in my heart, too, and make room for the growing family, the new relationships, and the increased responsibilities.

Then comes labour, like a shock wave. As the contractions come in quick succession, my directions allow me to widen my field of awareness and create some distance between the pain and me. Because I know that this pain is functional and not pathological, I try to react to it as little as possible. To ignore it is impossible. To eliminate it with the help of chemicals, besides being dangerous, is to deny myself the experience of feeling the work of nature. Why not live it, then, free from design or judgement?

From moment to moment, but above all at difficult times, I observe that my knowledge of the Alexander Technique gives me the possibility of choice: in this case, to resist or to accept. This insight helps me not to give in to panic when the pain threatens to engulf me. 'I let my neck be free, I receive these sensations, I let them come, I let them go.' I make good use of the pauses between contractions, and I collect myself physically and mentally, returning to that precious neutrality, that unmoving centre.

When the time comes for me to give up possession of the human being inside me, I loosen myself from the tensions in the upper part of my body, my neck, and my shoulders. I do not act; instead, I let it be, I let it open, I let it come.

Finally the child is there – despite her smallness, she is a heavy weight in my arms because she lets go of herself completely. I must now learn to hold her, to feed her, to bathe her. Again, the Alexander Technique is a source of strength: I pay attention as much to myself as to the child, and I do not freeze my shoulders or my lower back in an uncomfortable position. Released from the fear reflex, I do not grip my baby tight against me. Instead I support her – up along her body – and give her space and freedom.

With or without the Alexander Technique, labour and birth remain one of the most intense moments of human existence. Such an intensity is justified and welcome. The Technique is not a panacea, and it does not replace good sense. For me it is like a light that I send forth before me, a light that guides me as I move forwards. The Technique is also a mirror: when I am confronted with a problem, the Technique makes me face my own use instead, which soon helps me see the solution rather than the problem. Then it is up to me to allow the situation to evolve or not.

(Catherine de Chevilly teaches the Alexander Technique in Haute Savoie, France.)

DYSLEXIA

We have considered the question of emotions in depth. We have studied problems that are muscular or skeletal in origin. I hope that these discussions have helped you accept that it is utterly impossible to separate body and mind, posture and attitude, and physical sensation and emotional feeling. If this now seems logical and sensible to you, you will agree with me that it is also impossible to separate intellect and co-ordination.

Dyslexia, narrowly defined as the difficulty to recognize words and to read, has long been considered an intellectual problem, for which the solution is 'to concentrate'. In other words, the dyslexic learns how to concentrate, in order to become better able to read. Yet, despite his efforts of concentration, the dyslexic remains a slow reader. He is often obliged to re-read words, phrases, and whole passages several times, and never reads for the sheer pleasure of it. As well as his efforts of concentration, the dyslexic relies on a large arsenal of tricks and stratagems. For example, American children memorize the alphabet with the help of a song. Dyslexics can also learn the song; to the extent that they can sing it, they know the alphabet by memory, yet they are unable to recite the alphabet unless they sing it.

Current thinking about dyslexia, as exemplified by the work of Ronald D. Davis, author of *The Gift of Dyslexia*, sees it as a multi-faceted state of which a learning disability is just one aspect. Many of the other aspects are seen as positive, and include the dyslexic's ability to learn certain things much faster than non-dyslexics, a strong intuitive side, and mediunic and telepathic potential.

According to Davis, the dyslexic's use of tricks and ruses (such as singing the alphabet) closes off other avenues for learning. While providing a semblance of control and ability, the tricks actually lessen the dyslexic's capacity for the greater control of a normally functioning human being.

The dyslexic's tricks, concentration included, illustrate to perfection the Alexander principle of end-gaining. They achieve a specific goal at the price of making other, greater goals unachievable. The solution to a dyslexic's problems passes necessarily through inhibition: before he can do the right thing, he has to stop doing or prevent the wrong one. In other words, before he learns how to use his thinking well, he has to stop using it badly. Davis explains that dyslexia is a state of disorientation and confusion. It is aggravated by fatigue, malnourishment, and stress; dyslexics are more pointedly dyslexic when they are tired, hungry, or under pressure. Certain aspects of the therapy proposed by Davis are specific to the unique abilities of a dyslexic and need not be discussed here. One of his exercises interests us, though.

At some point in his re-education, the dyslexic stands on one leg while another person throws two objects at him, which he must catch with each hand. This re-trains the dyslexic's balance, enabling him better to prevent the disorientation that follows confusion. The re-education of the dyslexic according to modern practice, then, includes a kinaesthetic or proprioceptive element. The Alexander Technique is an extremely powerful tool for awakening, correcting, and refining proprioception, so it seems to me that it should be exceedingly useful in the treatment of dyslexia. However, the rôle of the Technique goes further than training 'the body', so to speak; after all, it is the inhibition of end-gaining – a psycho-physical process – that makes the changes in co-ordination possible. Inhibition, as we saw earlier, is also the key element in handling stress. Indeed, it redefines it, for if you react differently (or perhaps even not at all) to a stressful situation, it may cease to be a stress altogether. For a dyslexic, the absence of stress may entail the mitigation of the confusion and disorientation normally triggered by stress, and, consequently, the mitigation of the dyslexic symptoms that follow the disorientation. Dyslexics need therapeutic tools specific to their needs. The Alexander Technique cannot replace these tools, but it can certainly make their use easier.

Incidentally, my observations about dyslexia apply to all learning situations and intellectual endeavours. Let us call a dyslexic's response to stress 'abnormal'. A person whose reaction to stress is 'normal' also becomes disoriented and anxious under stress (passing an exam or doing a job interview, for example), only less so than the dyslexic. It is possible to have an 'ideal' reaction to stress, in which case the stress becomes just a stimulation. Just as the dyslexic can use inhibition to pass from 'abnormal' to 'normal', so can the ordinary person use it to pass from 'normal' to 'ideal'. Learning a foreign language, following the written instructions to operate an appliance, filling in tax return forms then all become easier and more pleasurable (yes, even filling in tax returns!).

IS THE ALEXANDER TECHNIQUE SCIENTIFIC?

The Alexander Technique has always earned the support of part of the medical and scientific community. Early on in his teaching career, Alexander was championed by several doctors; indeed, it was thanks to the encouragement of a prominent surgeon in Sydney, Dr J.W. Stewart McKay, that Alexander finally decided to quit his native Australia and try his luck in the capital of the Empire in the spring of 1904. (Alexander never went back to his birthplace, spending the rest of his life in Britain and the United States.)

Alexander was eminently successful in London. In 1937, a group of nineteen doctors published a letter in *The British Medical Journal*, inviting the scientific community to study his technique in depth and exhorting medical schools to incorporate it in their curriculum. The neurologist Sir Charles Sherrington, Nobel Prize for Medicine or Physiology in 1932, knew Alexander and appreciated his work; he had mentioned it in one of his books, *The Endeavour of Jean Fernel*, which first appeared in 1946. George Coghill, the American biologist and naturalist, admired Alexander and wrote a substantial introduction to one of Alexander's books. In it, Coghill discussed the Primary Control and the similarities between Alexander's discoveries and his own scientific work. The South African Raymond A. Dart, lecturer in anatomy and physiology, known world-wide for his anthropological studies (including the discovery of *Australopithecus*), met Alexander, studied the Technique, and wrote extensively about it.

In 1973, the ethologist Nikolaas Tinbergen shared the Nobel Prize for Medicine or Physiology with Karl Lorenz. In his acceptance speech, Tinbergen – who was taking lessons in the Technique at the time – spoke at length about Alexander and his work. It was undoubtedly the Alexander Technique's finest moment in scientific circles.

Tinbergen characterized the Technique as 'an extremely sophisticated form of rehabilitation, or rather of redeployment, of the entire muscular equipment, and through that of many other organs. Compared with this, many types of physiotherapy which are now in general use look surprisingly crude and restricted in their effect, and sometimes even harmful to the rest of the body.[23] ... Although no one would claim that the Alexander treatment is a cure-all in every case, there can be no doubt that it often does have profound and beneficial effects... both in the mental and somatic sphere.[24]

Because of faulty sensory awareness, it is possible for us to be wrong in what we do, say, and think, however certain we may be of the rightness of our actions, words, and beliefs. When you understand and accept this principle, you lose your fear of being wrong, thereby becoming less vulnerable and more open-minded. The true scientific spirit is permanently in doubt of itself; the history of science is the history of abandoned certainties. Yet there are many men and women of science whose minds are not actually scientific, but rather dogmatic instead. These men and women find it difficult to give up some of their convictions, regardless of whatever evidence may question them. We all tend to believe that a certain fact is 'true' because it is 'scientific'; let us call such a fact a 'clinical truth'. Yesterday's clinical truth is today's source of astonishment, or even ridicule. A single example should suffice. Not long ago, homosexuality was considered both a disease and a crime (which in itself happens to be a patent contradiction – can someone really be guilty of a disease?)

In the 1940s, Alexander was the victim of a vitriolic attack in the South African medical press by Dr Ernst Jokl, who at the time was in charge of the country's programme of physical education. Alexander sued him and won a retraction and substantial damages. The trial upset Alexander as much as the attack itself. Several well-known members of the scientific and medical communities testified for the defence, including doctors and physiologists who, like Jokl himself, had not even a passing knowledge of Alexander's discoveries. Their views were based exclusively on their preconceived ideas. Men and women of science sometimes say demonstrably false things using scientific terms. People who speak such nonsense are sometimes in a position of authority. Blinded by their authority and by their technical vocabulary, the public is quickly convinced that what they say must be 'clinically true'.

Despite the support that the Technique has received from the scientific community over the years, it remains more or less marginal in the world of medicine and science. It is true that, in Britain, lessons in the Technique are available in several clinics on the National Health Service, and, in some cases, private health insurance companies reimburse private lessons in the Technique. Yet the attitudes typical of an Ernst Jokl are prevalent everywhere.

Is the Alexander Technique 'scientific'? Towards the end of his Nobel Prize speech, Tinbergen said the following: 'What then is the upshot of these few brief remarks about the Alexander treatment? First of all they stress the importance for medical science of open-minded observance – of "watching and wondering".'[25] Clear your mind of any ideas you may have about the word 'scientific' and undergo a true scientific experiment: take a series of lessons in the Alexander Technique, as did Nikolaas Tinbergen, and study the inner logic of the Technique with an open mind, as Tinbergen exhorted us to do. Observe the effects of the Technique on yourself and on others who study it. Then, thanks to the authority that experience and insight give you, you will be perfectly capable to answer, for yourself, the question whether or not the Technique is scientific.

Alison, 26, Researcher

A bit of a sloucher, I was encouraged to 'sit straight and look up' as a child, but, like most people, I had not the slightest idea how to do so without discomfort. At the time I attributed my incapacity to sit straight to a lack of willpower. Though I would have liked to have perfect poise, I had always been fairly clumsy, smashing a disproportionate quantity of crockery on the kitchen floor. And I was no good at school sports. I loathed the humiliation of aimless throw after dropped catch after missed tennis ball. I responded to my failures by striving not to bother, to rise above it, which made me even less aware of my body. I was uncomfortable in class, sitting on the bus, reading books, or playing the double bass or piano.

My piano teacher was the first person to introduce me to some of the principles of the Alexander Technique. She taught me to release some of the tension in my neck and shoulder muscles as I played, and I was soon more comfortable sitting at the piano than anywhere else. But it was another ten years before I collected the courage and the cash to invest in some Alexander lessons with a qualified teacher. I finally took the plunge when I was working in an office, spending a lot of time sitting at a computer. I felt stressed out and my right shoulder had become painful.

After the first lesson I felt very relaxed, but surprisingly tired. Over the next couple of days, I felt as if my body was rearranging itself. Muscles and joints I had never been aware of ached, as if they were just coming back to life after suspended animation. In the weeks that followed, this gradual release of blocked joints and knotted muscles continued gently, and I began to be much more aware of my body and much more comfortable in it.

My initial enthusiasm led me astray. Keen to put my new-found principles of movement into practice, I made the mistake of trying too hard, stiffening my neck and back in my attempt to stay 'up'. When someone at work kindly remarked how sorry he was to see I had cricked my neck (when in fact all I was doing was trying to 'think up'), I realized that not only could I afford to take the Technique more lightly, but I would actually have to be a lot less earnest if I was going to learn it at all. From then on I started being kinder to myself when I got it all wrong. And there were days when I just had to laugh. One summer's day, I was sitting cross-legged and very 'up' on the grass outside a pub, singing the praises of the Alexander Technique to my friends. I then stood up to buy a round of drinks and promptly fell flat on my face – my poor crossed legs had gone entirely to sleep.

My Alexander teacher promised me that sooner or later good co-ordination would come naturally to me, so that being 'up' would be more comfortable than slouching.

This was not so at first, and for a while I suffered from what my teacher called 'Alexander's gloom'. Later I realized that failure is impossible, for the very concept of success or failure does not apply in the context of Alexander lessons. You just begin wherever you are and see how you change as you learn. When I accepted that, my 'Alexander's gloom' lifted as mysteriously as it had settled.

As my physical confidence increased, I began to be interested in the process of walking down the street, climbing the stairs, or hitting a tennis ball without worrying much about the result. Paradoxically, the more absorbed I was in the process rather than the end, the better the result became. I discovered a new technique for coming down the side of a mountain, by 'lunging from monkey to monkey' – not very graceful but surprisingly fast! I also found a way of preventing seasickness by balancing my head on my shoulders as if it were a bowl of tea I did not want to spill.

I took weekly lessons on and off for two years, but even if I had taken just a couple of lessons, I would have learned a lot from them. I can still tie myself in knots and tangles in a difficult meeting at work, or when speaking in public, and I still suffer some pain in my shoulder if I am under a lot of pressure or if I have been carrying a nephew or niece in my arms. But I avoid most of the pain I used to have, and I am able to undo a lot of excess tension. I cope much better with stress and have more stamina. Since I pay more attention to process than I used to, doing most things is easier and more fun. My Alexander lessons have been a rewarding investment, for which I am deeply grateful.

CHAPTER 7
Sports and Exercise

THE BENEFITS OF WORKING INTELLIGENTLY

You may take up exercise or practise a sport for various reasons, perhaps to lose weight, to sharpen your innate competitive spirit, to prevent or cure disease, or simply to have a good time. Regardless of your motivation, however, you should keep one thing in mind at all times: no activity is ever healthy in itself; it may become so depending on how you carry it out. Any action – whether a simple gesture in daily life or a complex athletic skill – may be performed in many different ways. Some of these ways are efficient, elegant, and health-giving; others are inefficient, inelegant, and even harmful. With certain kinds of exercise and sport, the potential for harm is enormous. This is proven by the number of people who take up a sport in order to deal with backache, for example, only to find that the sport itself aggravates the problem.

There are various aspects to exercising: the choice of activity, the intensity, duration, and frequency of exercising sessions, the choice of partners and venues, equipment and clothing, and so on. All other things being equal, however, the one factor that will make your exercising healthy or unhealthy is the way you use yourself.

Briefly, good use entails the inhibition of habitual, end-gaining responses that trigger misuse, and the co-ordinated direction of the whole body. The co-ordination of the body is determined by the orientation of the head, neck, and back. Good use is an outlook in life, an attitude as well as a posture; to use yourself well is to use yourself intelligently.

In exercise and sport, as in all other endeavours, the means condition the end directly, and the ends condition the means indirectly. In other words, the 'how' determines the 'what', and vice-versa. If you wish to become fit and healthy, you will be moving away from your goal if you do anything that makes you unhealthy. This apparently redundant observation is less laughable than you may at first think. People who exercise and practise sports tend to end-gain to a degree that makes their actions harmful. The possibilities for going wrong, aside from performing an exercise badly, are endless, and include trying to overcome severe unfitness in too short a period of time, trying to lose weight too quickly, competing above your level, working out when you are injured, and so on.

When you exercise, what matters is not to work your body hard, but to work intelligently. This applies not only to your use, but to all decisions that you take regarding exercise. In all these decisions, the Alexander Technique may play a useful rôle. Inhibition, which is the cornerstone of the Technique, is the ability to say 'no' to the temptation of achieving unreasonable goals using unreasonable means – in effect, not giving in to the temptation of doing something that may harm you.

Inhibition and direction have universal applications; they should allow you to bring a measure of intelligent co-ordination to every situation. Nevertheless, in some situations it is almost impossible to use yourself well and 'think up', and it may be better for you to avoid such situations altogether. The design of a racing bicycle, for example, makes it difficult to ride and think up at the same time. (The life expectancy of competitive bicycle riders is 60 years. This means that it costs them fifteen to twenty years off their lives to achieve their athletic goals.) In some sports, such as weight-lifting, even the finest athletes suffer severe health problems, which is an indication that the requirements of the sport run counter to nature. If you watch a high-level weight-lifting competition on television, particularly after you have acquired the ability to look at the world with Alexander-like eyes, you may be shocked and perhaps even disgusted at how brutally the competitors misuse themselves.

When assessing a specific activity, it is sometimes difficult to determine how much misuse is inherent in the activity and how much is caused by the way you perform it. If you are experienced and well co-ordinated, you may be able to take up many sports without harm. At the same time, it is likely that, as you become better co-ordinated and more in tune with the workings of your organism, you may wish to limit your activities to those that enhance your well-being without unjustified risks. In other words, it is possible to lift heavy weights intelligently, but it is more intelligent not to lift them at all.

Alexander made a pertinent point about fitness and health in one of his books, saying that 'continual re-adjustment of the parts of the body without undue physical tension is most beneficial, as is proved by the high standard of health and long life of acrobats. It is a significant fact that the very reverse is the case with athletes, showing that undue muscular tension does not conduce to health and longevity.'[26]

We could elaborate this observation further and state that fitness is a multi-faceted condition, which includes co-ordination, flexibility, strength, endurance, and quickness of reflex. It is easy to neglect one aspect in favour of another. Some athletes, for example, do not stretch as much as they should. Weight-lifters sometimes neglect their endurance; some hugely built-up men would not last for ten minutes on a treadmill. A competitive weight-lifter may justify this by claiming that endurance does not play a rôle in his competitions, therefore his time is better spent working exclusively on lifting weights. From the narrow point of view of immediate results, this over-specialization is easy to understand, although difficult to accept. From the broader point of view of health and well-being, such an attitude is regrettable (as are all other manifestations of over-specialization). If you are tempted to invest your energies intensely in a single activity, keep in mind that cross-training has for a long time been considered to enhance an athlete's ability at his or her primary sport. After taking a year off from competitive basketball to devote himself to baseball, Michael Jordan – also a keen golfer – went back to basketball to win yet another title in spectacular fashion.

Through good use, a person may benefit from performing an activity that is ill-conceived, or limited in some way. All the same, certain activities allow, encourage or even demand multi-faceted fitness; others do not. Good acrobats embody all the aspects of fitness; good weight-lifters do not. Similarly, some activities allow, encourage or even demand the upward thought characteristic of good use; others do not. Good martial artists think up; indeed, their upward direction is not so much a mark of mastery as its very source. Racing cyclists, however accomplished, are more or less prohibited from thinking up because of the design of racing bikes, and because of the nature of their activities. A masterly cyclist succeeds despite his mis-direction, not because of it.

We may conclude from the above that it is preferable to seek all-round fitness with the help of one or more activities that allow and encourage you to co-ordinate your whole self in an intelligent manner – or, better still, that positively demand you to do so.

THE PRIMACY OF FORM

In sports and exercising, good use is synonymous with good style or 'form'. Form and fitness are two separate things. A racing cyclist may be fit, but if he does not find his form on the day of the race he will not perform to his own best. Fitness is measurable in kilos, heartbeats per minute, chest capacity, body fat content, the rate of cholesterol, and so on.

'It is the string that makes the collar, not the pearls.' Gustave Flaubert

In conventional wisdom there is often more convention than wisdom. 'Swimming is the best exercise,' health magazines proclaim. Yet no exercise is good in itself; it may be good, indifferent, or harmful depending on how you perform it. The photo opposite was taken during the 1986 World Swimming Championships, and it depicts five professional swimmers executing their craft in five wholly different ways. Look at the swimmer in the middle. His pelvis advances forwards, making him hollow his lower back. The ridges across his lower back indicate that the misuse of his body is habitual, rather than a momentary lapse caught by a snapshot. Look at the swimmer immediately below him: he curves his body in the opposite direction, sticking his bottom out. Both swimmers let their necks drop forwards slightly in relation to the spine, which makes them less aerodynamic; imagine a bird trying to fly with its head dropped. The dropped neck will make the swimmers less hydrodynamic once they hit the water as well. Look at the black swimmer in the bottom of the picture. Although there appears to be a straight line running through his body, his back is severely narrowed, as you can see by the deep furrow that runs along his spine. His arms and shoulders advance away from the back; the impression that we have is that the shoulders are disconnected from the back and belong instead to the arms. He, too, drops his head. Look now at the swimmer on the top of the photo. Although at first his form appears quite good, his head is far forwards of his spine, and his shoulders seem to belong to his arms, not his back. Look finally at the swimmer placed second from the top. His head leads, his body follows. His neck is a natural continuation of his spine; indeed, we can say that his neck belongs to his spine, not his head. His shoulders too belong to the back, not to the arms, and his pelvis belongs to the back, not to the legs. This is not to say that he will win the race; it only means that, unlike his fellow competitors, he swims with the best possible form, thereby enhancing his health and well-being.

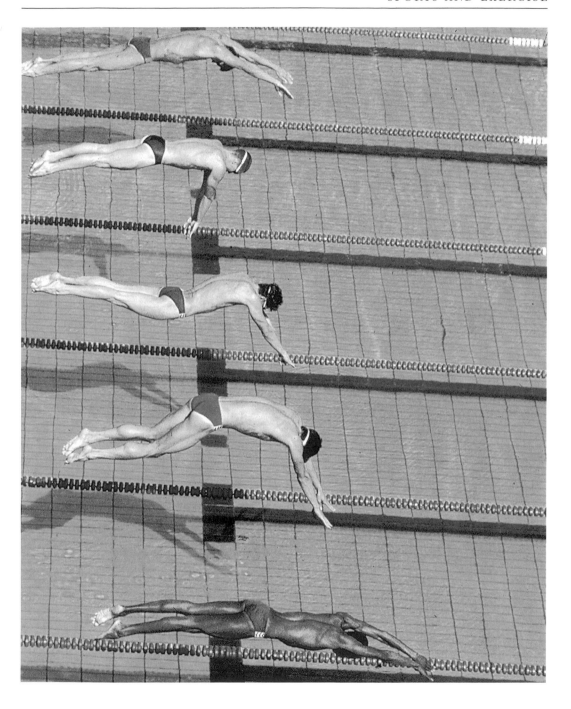

Form is a psycho-physical state that includes attitude and mood, and, unlike fitness, changes from moment to moment. Form contains an intangible element, more easily felt and observed than measured or described. When athletes talk about form, they soon start speaking in a manner that is lyrical, poetic, even metaphysical – the 'zone' is a term they often use.

Form and fitness do not depend directly upon each other. It is possible to be unfit in poor form, unfit in good form, fit in bad form, and fit in good form. Without any preparation, a well co-ordinated person – one who shows good form – could go for a long walk in the mountains without becoming fatigued. It is also good form that allows an old and slight woman to carry a large weight on her head, as is common in Africa, for example. This demonstrates the primacy of form over fitness in the matter of both endurance and strength.

Form and fitness may each perform a role in developing the other, although their interplay is unequal: form is the more powerful of the two. On the one hand, if you bring good form to your search for fitness you will *certainly* become fitter, and more quickly, than without it. On the other hand, fit people may *possibly*, but not necessarily, be better able to achieve good form. Fit athletes who do not show good form prove this point.

Good form, synonymous with good use, should take precedence over all other considerations. Aim not to run as fast as you can at any price, but as fast as you can while keeping good form. In the short term, this may cause your results to deteriorate. One fine booklet about running recommends the following: 'Do what comes naturally, as long as "naturally" is mechanically sound. If it isn't, do what is mechanically sound until it comes naturally.'[27] This is a play on two meanings of the word 'natural': according to the laws of nature, intrinsically right; and spontaneous, unpremeditated. You should cultivate what is intrinsically right ('natural') until it becomes reflex ('natural'), even if the sensations associated with what is mechanically correct unsettle you at first.

You may well run faster with habitual bad form than with inhabitual good form, but this may prove costly, since bad form increases the risk of accidents and injuries. In the long term, good form should guarantee optimal competitive results while enhancing your health and well-being.

In order to discuss the wish to win and its effects on an athlete's game, Alexander recounted an amusing anecdote about the tennis player W. H. (Bunny) Austin at Wimbledon. At one stage in the game, Alexander wrote, Austin 'was playing so badly he decided not to try to win the set but ... as soon as he had made that decision, he began to play up to his usual form. In consequence, he decided that now he would try to win the set after all, and immediately reverted to the indifferent play that had cause him "not to try".' Alexander, ever the provocateur, then concluded that 'it does seem sometimes as if human beings not only like to be fooled by others but are keen on fooling themselves.'[28]

Simply put, to go directly for an end (to win) causes a misuse of the self (the indifferent play), which makes the end unattainable. A good idea is to enter competitions wishing not to win, but to do your best, which may or may not assure you of a prize. Rod Laver, the great Australian tennis champion, seems to share this view:

You do the best you can. If you don't play your own game, you're going to lose it anyway. If you start to worry about the importance of the win before it happens, you're going to have yourself in a complete panic. You play the shots as you see them. That, and don't start wishing the shots to go in. When you start wishing, you are in trouble.[29]

Form requires a certain attention, and the participation of the conscious will that directs each gesture. For a well co-ordinated athlete, the awareness of his form is entirely salutary, and he may even have the impression that his form takes care of itself. This does not mean that his conscious will does not direct his form, but, rather, that it directs form harmoniously. When you first acquire a little awareness of your form, however, you may be struck – and discouraged – by how often you go wrong. It is easy to start feeling that every step, every dive, every throw is too far from an ideal of good form. You can then drive yourself crazy with the wish to be 'right', and with the awareness of being 'wrong'. Indeed, your very awareness of your 'wrong' steps causes you to go wrong, and, the harder you try, the worse things get.

The solution is for you to *allow* yourself to go wrong, and to observe what you do without judging yourself. Think not of 'getting it right' every time, but of widening your margin for error. Given the right conditions, you can have a lot of leeway in doing things supposedly 'wrongly'. If some constants of co-ordination are solid enough, there will be a degree of 'rightness' inherent in everything you do. In this case, some aspects of your performance will right themselves, and others will simply become unimportant. Sooner or later, your attention to form will cease to distract or discourage you, and will instead improve your results and increase your enjoyment of whatever you do.

The passage from adequate form to great form is almost inevitably awkward. The great British golfer Nick Faldo spent two years re-learning his technique early on in his career, when he was already succeeding professionally. To the dismay of his friends and admirers,

his competitive results deteriorated before he completely mastered his new swing. Afterwards, however, he climbed to the number one spot in the world rankings, proving that to master form is the surest way to achieve optimum competitive results.

SENSORY AWARENESS, HABIT, AND USE

Never take your form for granted – neither from moment to moment, nor in the long term. If you run a lap in good form, it does not mean that you will automatically run your next lap in equally good form. Similarly, if you find your form one day, there is no guarantee that it will stay with you tomorrow or the day after.

Two interconnected forces are at play here: faulty sensory awareness and habit. Most people have an imprecise idea of what they do and who they are. If you watch an exercise class, for example, you may see twenty different people performing the same exercise in twenty different ways. One participant may be twisting his neck, lifting his shoulders, hollowing his back, clenching his jaw, and holding his breath, all the while believing (or, rather, feeling) that he is perfectly relaxed. This is faulty sensory awareness at work. Most people in our hypothetical exercise class are misusing themselves without knowing it. Indeed, we can state as axiomatic that most people, most of time, suffer from faulty sensory awareness.

The only sure way of improving your sensory awareness is to improve the way you use yourself; the better your use, the more accurate the feedback you receive about yourself. Some techniques, such as watching yourself in a mirror, may help you become better aware of how you perform your exercises. However, it is easy to look without seeing, in which case the mirror may well be useless. If you do not know what you ought to be looking for, or if you judge your appearance without the detachment of a clinical eye, to look in the mirror becomes an exercise in simple narcissism. This is true if all you say is 'I am beautiful' or 'I am ugly' when you watch yourself. However, if you observe, for example, that you lift your right shoulder when you turn your head sideways, your self-scrutiny becomes objective and eminently useful.

Habit is inextricably tied to sensory awareness. The mind has an innate tendency to seek out the stimulation of the new, which necessarily crowds out the old. Once we become used to something, we are likely to stop noticing it. Often it is only when a certain sound stops – the humming of a refrigerator, for example – that we realize that it was there all along. It is the same for our habits, which are for the most part invisible to us.

The way you use yourself determines the functioning of your organism, for good and for ill. Alexander called the unceasing influence of use upon functioning 'the universal constant in living' (using this expression as the title of his fourth, and last, book), and he once defined habit as a manifestation of that constant. Rather than controlling habit by acting upon it *directly*, he recommended working on use instead. Since habit is simply a manifestation of your use, to change your use will necessarily cause an *indirect* change in all your habits, including those associated with your form.

Ideally, you should direct your whole self the whole time, and bring an upward thought to your every activity. You think up and walk, think up and speak, think up and eat, think up and compete. If you are able to do so, every one of your actions contributes to your ever-greater well-being. Until you start thinking up in action, however, you need to take time off away from action in order to cultivate your upward thought.

In practical terms, this means taking time before, during, and after an exercise session to work on your use. It could be a few minutes lying on your back, for example, performing a series of well-executed monkeys, lunges, and whispered 'ah's', or even simply pacing steadily and turning your mind not to how far or how fast you are about to run, but how you want to use your head, neck, and back as you do it.

If you work out at a health club, it is extremely useful to take breaks from exercising to renew your upward thought; besides the procedures suggested above, you may also benefit from taking a few moments to watch other people working out. Most people misuse themselves badly when they exercise; watching them is essentially a lesson in what *not* to do. A few people, however, do show good form, and you should analyse and study their style, soak up their psycho-motor intelligence, and imitate their good use.

It is again useful to take a few moments at the end of your workout to renew your awareness of your form, by lying down or slowing your activity to the point where you can easily think up. Aim to finish your session with a clear feeling not that you have been working hard, but that you have been thinking up in action.

TENSION AND RELAXATION REVISITED

Good form is not a matter of relaxation, but of necessary tension. Watch people on the rowing machine at the health club. Almost always, an athlete of average co-ordination keeps his spine and neck too relaxed, so that he curves his back and lets his head flop backwards and forwards with each row. This makes his form less efficient, and the rower tries to compensate for it by over-tensing other parts of his body – his arms and shoulders, for example.

For him not to be over-tense, then, first he needs the right tension, in the right amount, for the right length of time, and in the right places. This includes the neck, which needs right tension to support the head properly.

What most people call 'relaxation' is really a form of collapse, and as such it is more a problem than a solution. Interestingly, it is often more difficult for a too-relaxed (or hypotonic) person, whether athletic or sedentary, to find his necessary tension than for a too-tensed one (or hypertonic) to redistribute his tension with intelligence.

Necessary tension is not a quantitative matter alone – 'enough' tension or 'enough' relaxation. It is not a matter of combining tension and relaxation either; just as a singer who sings in tune is not one who sings a mixture of notes, some too high and others too low, the well co-ordinated athlete is someone who shows no wrong tensions and no wrong relaxations. The amount of tension, its placement, and its timing all play a rôle in good form, but quality of tension is the greater determining factor. When an alert infant holds your hand, or wraps her arms around your neck and her legs around your waist as you pick her up, the quality of the muscle tone in her whole body – its texture, intensity, and distribution – is a good example of what you should aim for in your co-ordination. Her tone is supple, firm, elastic, and very much alive. An experienced, caring doctor handles clients with a similar touch, which leads them to open up to the examination. What determines the quality of this touch is not so much a bodily condition but an inner attitude of self-assurance, openness, and trust – in yourself and in others.

Necessary tension is more easily demonstrated than explained or described. Achieving it is a matter of some difficulty too. Imagine that I find your spine too slack. If I ask you to increase its tonus, you are likely to stiffen your neck and make your head immobile. If I then ask you to free your neck, you may well make your spine slack again. The two concepts of separation and integration are useful when seeking necessary tension. Ideally, there should be some degree of separation between certain body parts – for example, between the head and the spine, between the shoulders and the arms, between the arms and the hands, and so on. By separation I mean mobility; if your head is properly separated from the spine, you can move it easily (or let me move it for you), without disturbing the state of the spine.

However, all body parts need also to be fully integrated into a harmonious whole. Mobility on its own is not sufficient, and in the absence of integration it may well be harmful. The neck, for example, is simply a

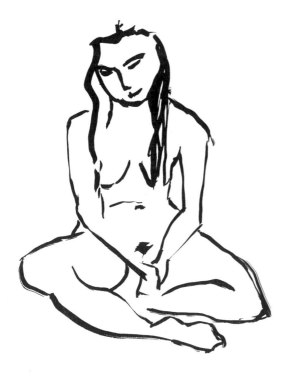

Relaxation is dispersal.

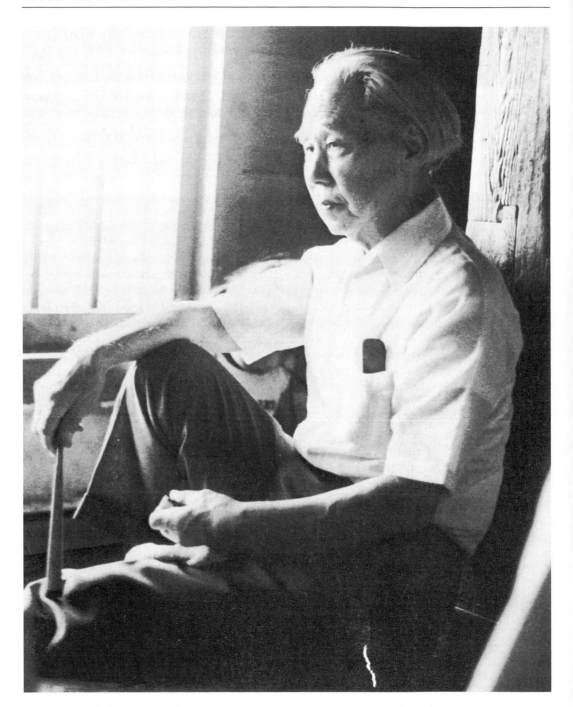

Containment is abundance. The aikido master Yukiyoshi Sagawa, aged 84.

continuation of the spine and should be integrated into it. Both the neck and spine have a high degree of suppleness, but this does not mean that they should be too supple, too relaxed, or too mobile. People often move their necks when they move their heads – as they look down at their feet, for example. It may be better to protect the unity between the neck and spine, and move the head without moving the neck. In other words, the neck and spine are integrated, and the head and spine are separated. The back and shoulders are integrated, and the shoulders and arms are separated. The back and pelvis are integrated, and the pelvis and legs are separated. In integration, there is necessary tension; in separation, there is the relaxation that is a side-effect of integration.

Necessary tension, the mark of good form, always involves the co-ordination of the whole body. It is the co-ordinated participation of every muscle group that ensures efficiency and success. 'Participation' does not entail active engagement. It could be that some muscle groups should remain completely disengaged as you perform your activity. But you may well need to use your brain actively to direct these muscle groups to remain passive, lest they tense up needlessly. In the words of Sir Charles Sherrington, a Nobel Prize-winning biologist who knew Alexander and admired his work, 'to refrain from an act is no less an act than to commit one'.[30] To command muscles to stay disengaged is as much an activity of the brain as to command others to become engaged, and an ideal balance between the two is the true meaning of co-ordination.

The body's mechanisms are so interconnected that muscle groups that seem to be unimportant or far removed from the focus of action may well play a crucial role in co-ordination and good form. Bud Winter, a great running coach with a string of world records

to his credit, says the following about testing sprinters over short distances: 'If [the sprinter] is any kind of athlete, he'll do [30 yards with a flying start] in three seconds. Then we talk it over and I tell him to have two things in mind when he runs it again – keeping his hands loose and his jaw loose. Invariably, he takes from one-tenth to two-tenths off his speed.'[31] This shows how the jaw and hands play a role in running, but the principle extends to *all* body parts in *all* activities. Some parts are more important than others, but no part is negligible. Some parts should be left loose, while others have to be brought into action. Even as a runner loosens up his thumbs, he must not allow his wrists and hands to be too relaxed and flop around; this would hinder the pumping action of his arms. The Alexander teacher and runner Malcolm Balk elaborates this point, among others, in his testimonial.

THE ALEXANDER TECHNIQUE AND RUNNING – MALCOLM BALK

I started running in 1975, after retiring from ice hockey, a sport I had played for the previous thirteen years. This was during the first running boom, and like many others I got caught up in the excitement and started running marathons. As a hockey player I had always accepted injuries as part of the game. So when I first experienced many of the common running problems – inflammation of the Achilles tendon, runner's knee, lower back pain, and so on – I felt they were all part of being a runner.

The other love in my life at that time was the cello, which I had great difficulty playing for any length of time without tension and discomfort. In fact, it was my desire to improve my ability to play the cello that led me to the Alexander Technique. As my lessons progressed, I felt I was on the threshold of discovering how to tap my potential and learn to overcome or avoid the obstacles that stood in my way. I decided to investigate the Technique in depth and to become a qualified teacher.

With that purpose in mind, in 1982 I moved to England, the 'land of the gods' – where Seb Coe, Steve Ovett, Dave Moorcroft, and Steve Cram lived and trained, and where F.M. Alexander had spent most of his life. For three hours every morning a group of thirteen students from all over the world would meet at the school run by the late Patrick Macdonald near Victoria Station. In some Alexander training schools, students are strongly advised to cease any vigorous activity until they have integrated the principles of the Technique sufficiently to prevent muscular effort from reinforcing existing patterns of misuse. I discussed this with Mr Macdonald, who gave me permission to keep running as long as he could ascertain that I was not doing myself any harm. I was grateful for the freedom to train, and found Mr Macdonald's watchful permission all the more reason to pay attention to how I was running.

Inspired by Coe's world-record 800-metre run in 1979, in which he had shattered the previous mark in an incredible display of effortless power, I had decided to move down from the marathon to the 800 metres. My training for the marathon had taken place mostly on the road. Now, as I trained for the 800 metres, I became a regular at the West London Stadium [since renamed the Linford Christie Stadium, in honour of the great sprinter]. I learned how to do intervals on the track, subdividing my runs into, say, four repetitions of 200 metres, each followed by a short rest period. Interval training allows the runner to train at a faster, more intense pace, yet as I trained the opportunity to repeat the cycle of injury, recovery, and new injury loomed large.

Fortunately, my Alexander training began to provide me with what we might call a kinaesthetic conscience. I began to be much more aware of myself as I went through my daily activities, from sitting at the table, to tying my shoes, to reaching for my pint (at least the first one!). I had been familiar with the saying, 'If you listen to the whispers, you won't have to hear the screams.' But up until I started learning the Technique, the idea of paying attention to the whispers seemed almost a contradiction to the "No Pain, No Gain" approach to running, to which I had subscribed wholeheartedly. Previously I, like many other runners, would be completely unaware of the warning signals which occurred when I trained. What is worse, when I was aware of the signs I ignored them: aches and pains, cold- and flu-like symptoms. My typical response, through what Alexander called 'stupidity in living', had been simply to run through them. Thanks to the Technique, however, I became ever less willing to overlook these signs or dismiss them as trivial or insignificant. This did not mean that I would stop running every time my knee twinged or my guts ached from the intensity of training or racing. Training and racing both require the athlete to tolerate a fairly high level of discomfort. It was more a matter of not letting my desire to achieve a particular goal cloud my judgement and ability to know when to back off and when to go on.

As I immersed myself in the teachings of Alexander, I started paying attention to what runners and coaches call 'form' and what Alexandrians refer to as 'use'. I made it an integral part of my running practice to monitor how hard my feet were hitting the ground, how much I tensed my shoulders, whether I was pulling my head backwards and shortening my spine, whether I was running smoothly or bouncing up and down, where my eyes were focused, and so on.

It has been said that the price of freedom is eternal vigilance. We could paraphrase the saying and state that the price of good form is eternal awareness. Elite marathoners tend to pay attention to sensory feedback that arises in training and competition – including sensations of discomfort, pain, and so on – while lesser runners tend to cope with the discomfort of their efforts by attempting to make the sensations disappear – for instance, imagining themselves relaxing on a beautiful beach. Runners call the first approach 'association' and the second, 'dissociation'. Association allows runners to hear the whispers and to make necessary adjustments before it is too late.

As a marathoner I had adopted what I considered to be an efficient running style, which I now describe as the 'marathon shuffle': a short stride with little or no knee lift and the tendency to land heavily on the heels. I would often pull my head back, and tended not to move my arms much. While this style allowed me to train for five marathons and complete all of them, it bore little resemblance to the fluid motion I saw in Coe or Ovett.

My coach at the time told me that if I was going to run the 800 metres I needed to improve my habitual form, which at the time was slowing me down. Running fast is a matter of stride length and stride frequency. In order to increase the length of my stride, I needed to learn how to run tall – how to 'keep the height', as my coach would put it. I remember another coach grabbing me by the hair and literally pulling me up in an effort to stop me from what he called 'sitting on my legs'. As my practice of the Alexander Technique improved – with its emphasis on lengthening, particularly the back – I learned to 'keep the height' without having to be yanked up and without fabricating a soldier-like posture that is in any case impossible to maintain. My ability to 'think up along the spine' made it easier to lengthen my stride, all the while

giving me more choice in my running: I was no longer a one-pace runner but could now call on several different gears which I would change to suit the circumstances.

Alexander saw that we can no longer rely on our instincts to guide us accurately in our activities. Faulty sensory awareness is all the more powerful for being intimately connected with our mental conceptions of how to do things. When I first started running, I thought that I ran with my legs – an idea which may seem so obvious as to be indisputable. Yet consider for a moment these words by the late Percy Cerutty, Australian Olympic coach: 'You run on the legs, not with them.' Alexander emphasized the orientation of the head to the neck, and of both head and neck to the back, as the key to effective movement. In harmony with Alexander's view, Cerutty saw leg movement as a natural extension of what occurs in the torso. Runners who run with their legs often tend to neglect what happens above the hip joint, and end up doing more than is necessary in order to compensate for their neglect. For example, if a runner pulls his head into the spine or allows it to roll from side to side he unwittingly increases the load and work of the legs.

To get a rough idea of why the poise of the head plays such an important role in good running, take a ten-pound weight (the approximate weight of the head) and hold it out at arm's length, better to appreciate the pull it is capable of exerting on your body. Now imagine your neck muscles straining with the effort of pulling that weight into your spine as you run. When you think of the hundreds and thousands of miles many runners log in a year, you can see how this problem would be something that should not be dismissed lightly.

When I first started running marathons I had no idea how useful my arms could be. I tended to hold them stiffly, yet – in the belief that 'relaxation is good' – with wrists so loose that my hands flopped about. I now know that my arms can support and energize my legs through their connection with my back, almost as if I were a quadruped. At times the arc of my arms is larger (when I sprint or climb hills) and sometimes smaller (when I run slowly on level ground), but in every case the potential for movement must remain active and alive. And my wrists need to remain toned, not floppy, in order to reduce my tendency to tighten my shoulders, thereby limiting the contribution my arms ought to make, especially when I am tired or need help changing gears.

The leg action of runners who run with, rather than on, their legs often lacks the fluidity, circularity of action, and smoothness we see in ten-year old girls (who are generally good natural runners), or in an accomplished runner whose full body is engaged in running. Runners who run with their legs push the pelvis into the legs, which increases the pressure on the lower back. They bounce upwards rather than rolling forwards, and pound into the ground rather than running over it, thereby contributing to the myriad lower leg problems that plague runners at all levels. They tend to focus on contracting their legs instead of releasing them, especially when trying to run more quickly, thereby forcing muscles to work against each other. 'The mind, drilled and grilled to wrong concepts, reacts against itself,' Cerutty wrote. 'The result is that as the athlete tries hard, the power exerted is transferred to his antagonistic muscles and the harder he exerts his power ... the more his brakes pull on.'[32]

When the running bug really bit me, I remember feeling that enough was never enough. If only I did more mileage, speed work, stretching, weights, and so on, I would run faster and achieve a goal sooner. This led to a phenomenon which affects many runners – I call it the Law of Diminishing Returns. You put in more and more to get less and less in return. For me, this meant increasing my mileage in the hope that it would lead to an improvement in my marathon time. Instead of better times, it resulted in more injuries and colds, and less enjoyment.

On the subject of marathons, an oft-aired view illustrates how different Alexandrian thinking is from received wisdom. The human body, the cliché goes, is not meant to run marathons; proof of it is that the first man to run a marathon dropped dead upon arrival. As the (possibly apocryphal) story is told, the soldier who ran to Athens to announce the defeat of the Persians by Miltiades in 490BC died after delivering his news. Yet the tale also includes an all-important detail: the soldier ran in full armour, after the heat of the battle. In one of his books, Alexander commented on Dorando Pietri, an Italian marathoner whom race officials helped across the finish line in the 1908 Olympic Games. Fatigued and probably dehydrated, Pietri staggered backwards as he approached the finish line. Alexander called him a magnificent athlete, and pointed out that, had Pietri known how to direct his use in times of stress, he would have oriented his head forwards and upwards, not backwards, and would have staggered towards the finish line, not away from it. Alexander's view on running marathons is simple: if you wish to push yourself to the limits of human endurance, make sure you know how to direct yourself in the best possible manner.

The finish line in every race presents an interesting study in end-gaining. As they approach it, runners give up any pretensions of poise or style. The uncontrollable urge to beat your opponent or shave a few seconds off your time sparks a response more akin to someone being attacked by a swarm of bees than to the poetry in motion we see in great sprinters such as Carl Lewis or Marie-José Perec. The head is thrown back, neck muscles become taunt with effort, the jaw is tightly clenched, the shoulders are raised up by the ears, and the arms flail frantically. What thrill there is in victory! But how fast can you really run when you so misuse yourself? In major competitions like the Olympics, the winner is often the runner who maintains the poise of his or her head right through the tape, as if there were no finish line.

Indeed, in every aspect of running the absence of a finish line makes for a useful metaphor. As head coach of the track and cross-country team at Concordia University, Montréal, I spend a lot of my energy convincing young athletes that they do not have to set a new personal best in every race in order to improve, and that trying to force improvement only leads to injury and burn-out. This can be a hard sell, particularly with runners who have experienced early success and expect this trend to continue unabated. One can only hope that they will not have to listen to too many screams before they tune in to the whispers.

Having learned to listen to the whispers, I myself have not suffered a single serious injury in my career as an 800-metre runner. Paying attention to my use has not hindered my performances in any way. On the contrary: for a while, I held the Canadian 1,500-metre record for the sub-master age group (from 35 to 40 years old).

But my greatest debt to Alexander goes beyond being healthy and winning races. 'The characteristic note of true happiness,' he wrote, 'is struck when the healthy child is busily engaged in doing something which interests it.'[33] Thanks to Alexander, I have maintained a healthy, child-like interest in running over twenty-two years – years of discovery and pleasure, but above all of happiness.

MODELS OF INTELLIGENCE

Imitation – a deep source of learning and growth, and an indispensable tool in human relations – is an ever-present phenomenon, even when you are not aware of it. As children, we imitate our parents, siblings, teachers, and colleagues. As adults, we look up to successful men and women. Often without meaning to, we allow ourselves to be influenced by people with strong personalities. Unconsciously, we end up imitating some aspects of their behaviour, including character traits that we may objectively find distasteful.

It is beneficial, therefore, to become aware of the mechanisms of imitation and to use them constructively. From the perspective of the Alexander Technique, a good model is not somebody who is prominent or successful, but, rather, a person who uses himself well. When I first took up ice skating, I watched closely a four-year-old child who was just beginning to skate, and who was a paragon of good use, his enormous head deliciously balanced on top of his little neck. Some older boys whizzed confidently by, but their bodies were contracted and distorted by the over-eagerness of end-gaining. We could say that the little boy skated 'badly', but, relative to his technical level, his style was perfect. Although he went carefully and slowly around the rink, he was a better teacher, for me and for everybody else, than the faster, more cocksure kids.

If what you imitate in a model is his or her good use, you need not limit your choice of model to people in your chosen field. For example, if you are a keen swimmer, you can improve your form not only by emulating accomplished swimmers, but also by learning from runners and golfers, dancers and musicians, other men, women, and children, and even animals. In effect, you would gain more from imitating a cat or a horse in motion than from imitating a swimmer who end-gains and uses himself badly.

Some constants of co-ordination apply to every human being and to every human endeavour. The healthy aspects of a great runner's style, for example, are equally healthy for all runners, independent of their sex, age or morphology. In addition, these aspects are equally good for playing tennis, walking, or just standing and waiting for a bus. Indeed, because these constants of co-ordination apply universally, you can improve your ability at sports and games while you sit, stand, walk, or even sleep, provided that you cultivate good form in all of these activities.

Once you really start to appreciate how universal the constants of good co-ordination are, you will find it increasingly enjoyable to watch great athletes at play, even if you do not practise their specific sports. The first impression of American football is that it is a brutal sport founded on sheer end-gaining, yet the best football players are models of intelligence and good use. Joe Montana, former quarterback of the San Francisco 49ers, is a case in point. On the eve of a tribute to Montana in which his No. 31 was retired, a number of players and coaches discussed his athletic prowess. Listening to them, we get the impression that they are talking about the principles of the Alexander Technique as embodied in the ultimate player.

Montana's career, both in college and as a professional, got off to a slow and doubtful start. According to George Young, the New York Giants' general manager, 'A lot of people worried about him because he didn't have big legs and a big arm.'[34] However, we can easily argue that the notion of an 'ideal' arm or hand is misleading. Heinrich Neuhaus wrote the following about pianists, but his observations apply equally well to athletes, and to men and women in ordinary occupations:

> Small hands with a small stretch have quite obviously to make much greater use of wrist, forearm and shoulder, in fact the whole of the 'hinterland', than large hands, particularly large hands with a large stretch … Sometimes this is just why gifted people with small and difficult hands have a better understanding of the nature of the piano and of their 'pianistic' body, than the large-handed and broad-boned.[35]

In short, the athlete whose throwing arm is unexceptional has an added incentive for using his whole arm in a manner that is intelligently co-ordinated with the rest of the body, thereby turning his perceived drawback into an advantage. Bill Walsh, Montana's coach at the 49ers, dispelled the notion that Montana could not throw. 'Because his delivery is not a flick of the wrist like Terry Bradshaw's, they think it's not strong,' he said. Walsh's remark about Montana's not flicking his wrist indicates that he used instead his entire arm, in harmony with the rest of his body.

Walsh also commented about Montana's ability to throw under any number of circumstances. 'He throws on the run while avoiding a pass rush, and he does not have to be totally set. He is not a moving platform like some others who are mechanical and can only do well when everything is just right.' To throw a football, a quarterback requires great stability, hence the 'platform' attitude of some players. As Walsh describes him, Montana displayed latent resistance *and* latent mobility – two hallmarks of good co-ordination – and put both into action separately and together, as needed, which made him more effective than earthbound players.

Montana's co-ordination was superb. From the perspective of an Alexandrian observer, however, what was even more interesting was his ability to keep his cool in extremely stressful game situations, and to time his moves to the advantage of the whole team. 'His gift as a quarterback,' noted sports journalist Lowell Cohn, 'was not so much his raw athletic ability, but his unflappable poise … Montana refused to throw a pass until precisely the right moment.' A former colleague, 49ers' guard Randy Cross, once said of him, 'He's rather detached. It's like he's able to do it in the third person.'

Montana's calm was a manifestation of his ability to *inhibit*: to withhold consent to an unintelligent reaction that may come too soon, too strongly or too weakly, or too eagerly. Indeed, his co-ordination and his powers of inhibition are one and the same. Joe Montana was a great athlete because he was extraordinarily intelligent on the field. If you decide to fashion your athletic self after him, you risk failure by copying his co-ordination without acknowledging the vital intelligence behind it. We tend to honour the intelligence of a scientist, a writer or a statesman, while envying an athlete's prowess or brawn. Yet there is no separation between the mind and the body, that is to say, between all that is physical and all that is mental. In one of the matches of the 1996 World Series, Greg Maddux of the Atlanta Braves played magnificently. After the match, Leo Mazzone, the Braves' pitching coach, said, 'Nobody can keep up with his [Maddux's] thinking processes.'[36] When talking about the NBA, Oscar Robinson, the distinguished basketball pioneer, said that 'the ability to think on the court'[37] was missing from the game as played today, in comparison with his times.

The outer characteristics of good form, as represented by Joe Montana, are the harmonious co-ordination of the whole body, the presence of necessary tension and its consequent relaxation, and the right balance between resistance and mobility, and between integration and separation. The inner roots of good form, superbly embodied by Montana, are the 'thinking processes': the well-directed, unflappable psycho-physical intelligence that makes sport a joyous celebration of life.

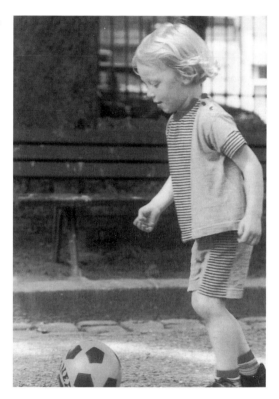

CHAPTER 8

The Performing Arts

TWO PERSONALITIES

It is Sunday night; while flicking through the television channels, you happen upon a classical music concert. A symphony orchestra plays a piece you do not recognize. Several cameras, strategically placed, allow you to watch all sections of the orchestra in turn – strings, woodwinds, and percussion, all directed by a lively conductor who needs a haircut. You put the remote control aside, and settle down to watch a fascinating lesson of virtuosity, of movement and posture, of concentration, musicianship, and professionalism. Little by little, your attention is caught by the particular sight of two young violinists who share a music stand. The cameras carry on showing the whole orchestra in alternation, but now you wait impatiently for the moment when the cameras focus on these two strikingly different players.

The violinist on the left – let us call her Heather – never stops moving, her back slightly rounded, her head drawn towards the music stand, her forehead wrinkled with intent. Her violin goes up and down with each stroke of the bow. Her head too moves with her violin; her long hair falls on to her face, and she throws her head back every two or three measures in order to see the music better. Her playing is full of energy, emphatic, insistent. You find her delightful. Indeed, you soon catch yourself moving your head in tandem with hers to the beat of the music, as

if you were making music yourself. You have become an active participant in the concert and take much pleasure in it. Yet, after a while you start noticing that a little tension in the back of your neck is beginning to nag you. Music-making, you tell yourself, is very tiring.

The violinist on the right – let us call her Marjorie – plays so differently from her stand partner that you have trouble believing that they are performing the same piece. She sits near the edge of the chair, her back straight, her head nearly immobile. Her violin does not move either; even the most vigorous bow strokes do not disturb her remarkable aplomb. When you look at Marjorie, you have the impression that her arms are wholly independent of the rest of her body. Her face is relaxed too. At first you find Marjorie a bit stiff, cold even, and certainly not as interesting as Heather. Soon, however, you realize that she plays with more than a little elegance. Her gestures, economical and sure, remind you of the gymnasts you saw during the last Olympic games. The young woman's comportment is so dignified, her playing so well directed, that you find yourself watching her with increasing admiration. You now notice that, for all her stillness in motion, her eyes burn with passion. At last you are hypnotized by the strength and beauty of her playing, and the music she is performing seems uncommonly powerful to you. The tension in the back of your neck has gone.

TO INTERPRET, TO TRANSMIT

Heather and Marjorie share a single characteristic: they both play the violin. Yet there could hardly be two more distinct human beings. They are distinct in thought and gesture, attitude, musical interpretation, and everything else. Heather wastes her energy. She uses too much effort to play the violin; more precisely, she mis-directs her efforts, thereby bringing about the constant up-and-down movements of her head and violin. These movements make her technique unreliable; they affect her bow arm, causing her unwittingly to press too hard on some notes and too lightly on others, and her left hand as well, making her intonation and her changes of hand position uneven. Her rhythm is irregular, too; because of her excitement, she tends to hurry and play ahead of her colleagues. At the end of each concert she is fatigued; at the end of the concert season she suffers from backache; at the end of a few seasons she begins to suffer from tendonitis, which may one day threaten her career.

Marjorie's technique is faultless. Her intonation and rhythm are both even. She is able to give each note the same sound, the same articulation, the same vibrato. Because of this ability, she can choose to change the musical sense of a note or phrase, giving it more or less weight, making it more or less interesting, according to the exigencies of the composer, or the instructions of the conductor. Her choices, then, are all based on musical judgement, rather than being pre-determined or limited by technical ineptness, as in Heather's case. Marjorie watches the conductor with unwavering attention, yet her watchfulness does not distract her from paying attention first and foremost to her own playing. She keeps her cool even when the conductor moves in a manner that is inelegant and unclear. We could say that Marjorie plays well even when the conductor conducts badly; generally, she does not let external events disturb her inner poise. At the end of a concert, she is full of energy. Her back does not hurt, despite the long orchestra tours with their endless rehearsals and uncomfortable chairs.

These two imaginary violinists illustrate several principles of the Alexander Technique. They each have their way of moving, of working, of expressing themselves as human beings and as artists. Simply, each uses herself in an individual manner. Several aspects characterize the use of the self: the expenditure of energy, the balance between tension and relaxation, the economy and elegance of gestures, and many others. Synonymous with co-ordination, a musician's use determines her technical ability, her dexterity or awkwardness, and her sound quality. The well co-ordinated musician plays with ease and lightness. She sight-reads an unfamiliar score without fear and learns new pieces quickly. She has a good muscular memory, thanks to which she remembers phrases, passages, and whole pieces easily, and retains the instructions of her teacher or her conductor. A well co-ordinated musician is likely to suffer fewer health problems than her badly co-ordinated colleague. Too much effort, tension, and fatigue usually lead to muscular and skeletal problems such as tendonitis, carpal tunnel syndrome, arthritis, bursitis, and so on.

The use of the self, then, affects the functioning of a musician, her technical abilities, and her health and well-being. However pertinent, our observations about use and functioning would be incomplete if we limited them to all that appears to be 'physical' in a musician's life. It is impossible to isolate the physical components of somebody's use from the mental ones. To each gesture corresponds an intention, and to each action a thought. What animates a free gesture is a conception that is also free. What makes Heather and

Marjorie contrasting, or even opposing musicians, is not their posture, but their attitudes, towards the violin, towards music, and towards themselves.

In music, as in all the arts, there is something magical, sacred, and exalted. I believe that, ideally, the rôle of a musician should be to reveal to the public the exaltation of which the work of art is an expression. When Heather makes music, she becomes so excited that she ends up drawing the attention of the public not towards the work of art, but towards herself. Her style of playing turns out to be costly for herself, for her public, and, ultimately, for the work of art.

Nadia Boulanger, the great French teacher of composition and music theory, spoke of the difference between interpreting and transmitting. When a musician interprets a piece of music, she focuses her light on herself. When she transmits it, she focuses it on the work of art. Marjorie uses such means in her playing – which is economical, well-directed, and detached, in the best sense of the word – so that she transmits to the public the intentions of the composer as revealed in the score, allowing the public to listen not to Marjorie's playing, but to the greatness of the work of art. It is one of the great paradoxes in an artist's life: to allow the work of art to shine in all its splendour, the artist must efface herself; yet, to efface herself, she needs to be intensely aware of her own self.

UNIVERSALITY AND INDIVIDUALITY

An Alexander teacher comparing Heather and Marjorie would quickly note that, as she becomes exalted in performance, Heather end-gains and misuses herself, while Marjorie inhibits her own excitement and uses the necessary means to reveal to the public the exaltation inherent in a musical work. Marjorie's attitude is characterized by self-restraint and detachment, both of which are inseparable from a certain co-ordination, technique, and sound quality. A musician who decides to stop end-gaining and misusing herself may need to abandon habitual gestures and ideas, such as those of Heather, to embrace new and different ideas, of which Marjorie is an exemplar.

This is not to say that all musicians should play in the same manner. It is possible for each of us to express our individuality despite using means that are universal. Alexander liked to say that individuality is simply a habit, which can be changed and transformed. At the end of the transformation, you will still express your individuality, but differently from before.

If you study the performances of several musicians who use themselves well, you may be struck on the one hand by all that makes

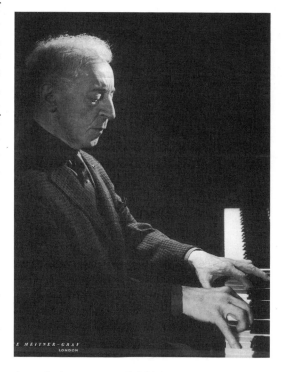

Artur Rubinstein 1887–1982.

them similar, from the point of view of co-ordination, posture, and movement, and on the other hand by all that makes each of them unique, from the point of view of sound quality, interpretation, and artistic outlook. The Swiss pianist Alfred Cortot and the Polish pianist Artur Rubinstein (both of whom lived for a good part of their life in France) had unique temperaments, convictions, and habits of thought and gesture. Someone listening to one of Cortot's recordings would not for a moment mistake him for Rubinstein, and vice-versa, yet both of them used themselves at the piano in a similar fashion. The back was firm and pointed upwards, the neck was a natural extension of the spine, the head moving, but little and without disturbing the line between the neck and the spine. All their gestures were discreet, economical, and powerful. Many other great pianists use themselves in such a manner. We may well say that master musicians are, for the most part, individual flowerings of a universal life force.

An artist's journey towards the Alexandrian ideal – which for a musician implies a change from interpreting to transmitting – is not without difficulties. Because of faulty sensory perception, a musician whose use is not natural is not aware of what he does. To become aware may well be upsetting. To feel tensions and misuses accurately for the first time may give the pupil the impression that he or she has suddenly become more tense than before. Musicians spend long years cultivating their habits of music-making. Habits are normally quite stubborn; habits developed in a conscious and disciplined manner over many years are even more obstinate. On top of that, a musician's habits are not simply physical or psycho-physical; they also contain an aesthetic and

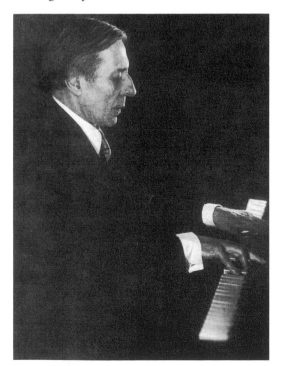

Alfred Cortot 1877–1962.

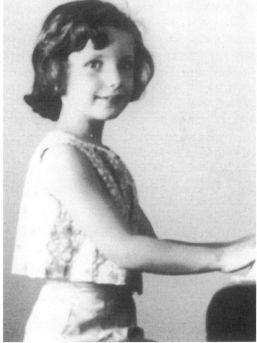

Annie, aged six.

professional component. In short, a musician has invested himself fully in his habits, and identifies fully with them. (This point is valid for all people who have cultivated similar habits in the course of their professional training.) To succeed in his self-transformation, a musician needs to work in a particular manner.

'A person who learns to work to a principle in doing one exercise,' wrote Alexander, 'will have learned to do all exercises, but the person who learns just "to do an exercise" will most assuredly have to go on learning to "do exercises" *ad infinitum*.'[38] Let us establish a series of factors which, taken together, create the working principle to which Alexander refers.

WORKING TO A PRINCIPLE

The principles and procedures of the Alexander Technique apply to all areas of musical activity, from technique, sound production, and interpretation, to daily practice, rehearsal routines, and the mitigating of stage fright and health problems. My first book, *Indirect Procedures: A Musician's Guide to the Alexander Technique* (Oxford University Press, 1997) discussed in detail the applications of the Technique to music-making. Here, I propose to highlight a few of the points of that book, in particular those concerning a musician's daily practice. (Although these observations are addressed to an imaginary musician reader, I should like to think that non-musicians could benefit from studying them too.)

1. When considering any problem ('technical' or 'musical', 'physical' or 'mental'), always keep in mind that, as a human being, you are individual and indivisible in all your actions. Carrying a cello up four flights of steps may be a more eminently physical activity than reading a musical score, but both are activities involving your whole being. Your daily practice may seem to you mostly a matter of training your body, yet there never exists a separation between body and mind. Sir Charles Sherrington, the Nobel Prize-winning biologist, wrote that 'the formal dichotomy of the individual [into "body" and "mind"] ... which our description practised for the sake of analysis, results in artefacts such as are not in Nature.'[39] Think of your daily practice not as a matter of training the body, but of restoring and refining the connections that exist ideally between body and mind.

2. No exercise is intrinsically healthy; it may become so according to the way you execute it. Over-eagerness, doubt, hurry, confusion or indifference can all stop you from performing an exercise properly. Even as you practise a simple finger exercise, a scale or an arpeggio, your mental attitude will determine whether or not the exercise is beneficial. Since you risk harming yourself by badly executing an exercise, have a clear mental picture of what you are trying to accomplish, and how you can best accomplish it. Approach every task in your practice with clarity of mind, imagination, and good humour. Contrary to what many musicians believe, 'concentration', depending on how you define it, is not necessarily the best frame of mind for the purposes of daily practice. To concentrate may mean to organize and co-ordinate a series of aspects around a central point. This was the original meaning of the word: a number of circles that share a centre. To some people, however, to concentrate has become, in practical terms, to isolate some aspects and eliminate others. Defined in this second way, 'concentration' is a state to be avoided rather than sought. It is easy to tell

when a musician is 'concentrating': he gazes into space without blinking, constricts his breathing, and stops speaking or listening. We could also call this 'self-hypnosis'. Trance-like conditions have their uses, but to co-ordinate yourself you need to quicken your conscious mind, thereby increasing your awareness of yourself, of others, and of the environment around you. When you become aware, you will not find it difficult to think of several things at the same time, in an orderly and constructive manner. You can think of your head, neck, and back as well as your bowing arm and your left hand, the evenness of your rhythm, the beauty and strength of your sound, your playing partners, and much more besides. Let us call this state 'awareness', and a state of unbreathing, unblinking stiffness 'concentration'. The mind that is aware can concentrate; the concentrated mind is often unaware. As you practise, then, *be aware*, and keep concentration at bay.

3. You engage your whole body whenever you perform a gesture, however small. When you play an open string at the cello, your head, neck, torso, and legs all play a rôle in determining how well you use your bow arm. If your back is not stable, for instance, you risk unbalancing your trunk as you draw your arm across the string, and tightening your neck and shoulders to compensate for that loss of balance. Needless to say, this would affect your ability to use your arm freely. Indeed, your primary consideration should be not your limbs (as you play or conduct), or your lips, tongue, and jaw (as you sing or play a wind or brass instrument), but the ideal co-ordination of your whole self, which depends on the orientation of your head, neck, and back. The biologist George Coghill wrote in an introduction to one of Alexander's books,

in my study of the development of locomotion I have found that in vertebrates the locomotor function involves two patterns: a total pattern which establishes the gait; and partial patterns (reflexes) which act with reference to the surface on which locomotion occurs ... Now the reflexes may be, and naturally are, in harmony with the total pattern, in which case they facilitate the mechanism of the total pattern (gait), or they by force of habit become more or less antagonistic to it. In the latter case they make for inefficiency in locomotion ... Mr Alexander, by relieving this conflict between the total pattern, which is hereditary and innate, and the reflex mechanisms, which are individually cultivated, conserves the energies of the nervous system and by so doing corrects not only postural difficulties but also many other pathological conditions that are not ordinarily recognized as postural.[40]

Coghill's 'mechanism of the total pattern' is the orientation of the head, neck, and back that Alexander called the 'Primary Control'. Ideally, the total pattern (hereditary and innate, in Coghill's words) should take precedence over all the partial patterns (individually cultivated). In short, every localized action – the activity of limbs, hands, and fingers, and of lips, tongue, and jaw – should be executed in harmony with the co-ordination of the head, neck, and back.

The defining characteristic of an ideally co-ordinated person is not relaxation, but *necessary tension* – the right kind of tension, in the right amount, at the right place, and for the right length of time (*see* Chapter 2).

4. If you use your left arm poorly, your right one will suffer, and vice-versa; let us call this 'bilateral transfer'. If you use one of your legs poorly, both the other leg *and* the two arms will suffer; let us call this 'quadrilateral transfer'. Bilateral and quadrilateral

transfer can be a force for good too; if you use your right arm well, your left one will benefit.

When executing every exercise, then, make sure that you are engaging all your limbs constructively, so that quadrilateral transfer can be a positive, not negative, factor. This does not mean that you need to move your arms and legs about whenever you use your fingers. Instead, make sure that you are not unduly contracting or collapsing any limb, and that every limb is well connected to the back.

5. 'The musician's bible', said the great conductor and pianist Hans von Bülow, 'begins with the words: "In the beginning there was rhythm."'[41] Good rhythm improves the way you use yourself, at the same time that good use improves rhythm; they feed each other. Breathing, circulation, love-making, and locomotion all demonstrate that healthy functioning is naturally rhythmic.

Perfect rhythm includes precision, but also energy, dynamism, and impetus – what musicians usually call *forward motion*. Forward motion is part of the quality in music that makes you want to tap your foot or pretend that you are the conductor. Speaking of the rhythmic element in the pianist Sviatoslav Richter's playing, Heinrich Neuhaus quotes Goethe: 'You think that you push but you are being pushed.'[42] Forward motion makes music *compelling*, and it adds a liveliness to rhythmic discipline that is lacking in mere metronomic precision.

It is practically impossible to benefit from an exercise if you do not execute it rhythmically. Therefore, perform every exercise, however simple or complex, with the greatest rhythmic precision and forward motion.

6. Technique has often been equated with co-ordination, and co-ordination with the ability to play fast notes. Speed and accuracy may be important *aspects* of technique, but so are clarity, evenness, intonation, and many others. We hear it said of someone that he has 'great technique', but an ugly sound. This is a patent absurdity. Wilhelm Furtwängler, conductor of the Berlin Philharmonic from 1922 to 1954, wrote that 'technique must make free regulation of the rhythm possible, and go beyond this to influence the tone.'[43] Heinrich Neuhaus concurs: 'Work on tone is work on technique and work on technique is work on tone.'[44]

The musician with an ugly sound may have great dexterity, which is just one aspect of technique, but he does not have a great technique. A complete technique implies the ability to play *legato* and *sostenuto*, in a wide range of dynamics and articulations, in every imaginable colour. Good technique contains in itself the seeds of musicianship. If you practise 'technique' in isolation from 'music', you risk mastering neither. You could easily find that you can play a passage evenly as long as you keep it empty of all expressivity, but that you lose technical control as soon as you attempt to make the passage expressive. Therefore, never execute a gesture or a phrase without taking into consideration its musical character.

To sum up the above points, you should always practise with the whole of yourself. The essential elements are attitude, posture, intelligence, imagination, humour, self-awareness, necessary tension, bilateral and quadrilateral transfer, rhythmic precision and forward motion, and musical content. If you leave one of these out, practising could cause you more harm than good.

IN THE MUSIC WORLD

The Technique has for a long time enjoyed the enthusiastic support of many musicians, amateur and professional, classical and popular. In Great Britain, most music schools training professionals (such as the Royal College of Music, the Royal Academy of Music, and the Guildhall School of Music and Drama) have Alexander teachers in their faculties. In the United States, many of the best schools (including the Juilliard School in New York, and the Curtis Institute in Philadelphia) offer lessons and classes in the Alexander Technique, as do schools and conservatories in Germany, Holland, Switzerland, France, and many other countries.

The penetration of the Technique in the world of music is not limited to music schools. A number of great concert artists have made use of the Technique, including the guitarist Julian Bream, the pianist Radu Lupu, and the singers Barbara Hendricks and Renata Scoto. Sir Colin Davis, for a long time chief conductor and musical director of the Royal Opera House in London and currently principal conductor of the London Symphony Orchestra, generously agreed to write a foreword to my book, *Indirect Procedures*. In it, he related how Sir Adrian Boult, himself a celebrated British conductor, first encouraged him to take lessons in the Technique some forty years ago.

Amateur musicians may also benefit from studying the Alexander Technique. I have already mentioned my pupil Geneviève (*see* Chapter 4), who started cello lessons when she was in her forties. 'A cello teacher,' she wrote, 'once told me, during a summer course: "You will never be able to play the cello, as the extensions between your fingers are too limited." My trouble with finger extensions was in fact only one among many difficulties. I sought out the Technique, and,

six years after studying it steadily, I have an increasing mastery of instrumental technique, which opens my musical horizons.' I wish the teacher who once said to Geneviève that she would never play the cello could now see and hear her improvise at the cello, with greater inventiveness and freedom than many professionals. It is foolish for a teacher to make definitive assessments of a student who has never been given the means to develop his or her potential. A musician who learns to inhibit and direct uses herself so differently that she then appears more talented than before. This only disproves the earlier assessment, since talent is an unchanging attribute.

Musicians outside the world of classical music have also studied and supported the Technique; Paul McCartney (who collaborated with Dr Wilfred Barlow on a documentary about the Technique) and Sting are two of the best-known among them.

CINEMA AND THEATRE

In Chapter 1, I recounted how Alexander developed 'the work', as he called it, in the process of solving certain vocal problems that had threatened his theatrical career. From early on Alexander enjoyed great success as an actor, director, and teacher. Naturally, the theatrical community was the first group of people to become interested in the ideas of Alexander the pedagogue. He became director of the Sydney Dramatic and Operatic Conservatorium, a post which he held until he left his native Australia for London, where he lived until his death in 1955. On arrival in London, Alexander made himself known to the artistic community, and taught many of the great actors and actresses of his time, including Sir Henry Irving, Lily Brayton, and Viola Tree, as well as the playwright George Bernard Shaw.

In 1930, Alexander started training teachers of his Technique. At first, he had envisaged devoting part of the teachers' training to the preparation and performance of a theatrical play, which he would direct and present professionally to the London public. He abandoned this practice after a few years. Indeed, despite his great love for the theatre (and especially for Shakespeare), Alexander found himself so deeply involved with teaching that he finally had to give up his theatrical activities.

In the great British theatre schools of today, such as the Royal Academy of Dramatic Art and the London Guildhall School of Music and Drama, the Alexander Technique is taught as a matter of course. The Royal Shakespeare Company makes Alexander lessons available to its members. The Technique is equally taught in theatre schools in the United States, including the Juilliard School in New York and university departments across the country.

Phyllis Richmond (*see* below) teaches the Alexander Technique in the Theatre Division of Southern Methodist University (SMU) in Dallas, Texas, and at the Blair School of Music at Vanderbilt University in Nashville, Tennessee.

THE ACTOR AND THE CHARACTER – BY PHYLLIS RICHMOND

An actor on stage is really two people at once: the actor and the character, each with a unique rôle to play in making the performance happen. The character's consciousness is inside the play – he or she is the one to whom the play is reality, the one who feels the emotions, has the intentions, and executes the actions. The actor's consciousness monitors the process of bringing the character to life, makes sure the actor speaks loudly enough, finds the hot spot, registers laughter and waits for it to subside, adjusts blocking to compensate for a scene partner who has moved by mistake, checks for unnecessary tension and releases it, and so on. The actor's consciousness facilitates the character's consciousness, attending to the conditions that allow the actor to go about the work of playing the character and proceeding through the journey of the play.

You're trying to catch the Guvnor's manner and you aren't making a bad fist of it, but there are one or two things you haven't noticed. You're an acrobat, good enough to walk the slackwire, but you're tight as a drum. Look at the Guvnor: he hasn't a taut muscle in his body, nor a slack one, either. He's in easy control all the time. Have you noticed him standing still? When he listens to another actor, have you seen how still he is? Look at you now, listening to me, you bob about and twist and turn and nod your head with enough energy to turn a windmill. But it's all waste, y'see. If we were in a scene, you'd be killing half the value of what I say with all that movement. Just try to sit still. Yes, there you go; you're not still at all, you're frozen. Stillness isn't looking as if you were full of coiled springs. It's repose. Intelligent repose. That's what the Guvnor has. What I have, too, as a matter of fact. What Barnard has. What Milady has. I suppose you think repose means asleep, or dead.

Now look, my lad, and try to see how it's done. It's mostly your back. Got to have a good strong back, and let it do ninety per cent of the work. Forget legs. Look at the Guvnor hopping around when he's being Scaramouche. He's nippier on his pins that you are. Look at me. I'm real old, but I bet I can dance a hornpipe better than you can. Look at this! Can you do a double shuffle like that? That's legs, to look at, but it's back in reality. Strong back. Don't pound down into the floor at every step. Forget legs.

How do you get a strong back? Well, it's hard to describe it, but once you get the feel of it you'll see what I'm talking about. The main thing is to trust your back and forget you have a front; don't stick out your chest or your belly; let 'em look after themselves. Trust your back and lead from your back. And just let your head float on top of your neck. You're all made of whipcord and wire. Loosen it up and take it easy. But not slump, mind. Easy!

Suddenly the old man grabbed me by the neck and seemed about to throttle me. I jerked away, and he laughed. 'Just as I said, you're all wire. When I touch your neck you tighten up like a spring. Now you try to strangle me.' I seized him by the neck, and I thought his poor old head would come off in my hands; he sank to the floor, moaning, 'Nay, spare m'life!' Then he laughed like an old loony, because I supposed I looked horrified. 'D'you see? I just let myself go and trusted to my back. You work on that for a while and bob's your uncle; you'll be fit to act with the Guvnor.

'How long do you think it will take?' I said. 'Oh, ten or fifteen years should see you right,' said old Frank, and walked away, still chuckling at the trick he had played on me.

From *World of Wonders*,
by Robertson Davies

The late Canadian author was a keen student of the Alexander Technique. He wrote about his Alexander experiences in a foreword he contributed to a book of essays on the Technique titled *Curiosity Recaptured: Exploring Ways We Think and Move*, edited by Jerry Sontag and published by Mornum Time Press.

This double consciousness is filled with paradox. The demands of the external and internal realities may not be the same – for example, the actor may be playing an intimate moment of self-revelation that must be heard in the back of the balcony. The connection between inner and outer aspects of acting technique must be developed so that it becomes second nature for the actor to express inner reality in outer form.

The problem is that the act of performing creates tensions that can interfere with performance. Too often, the actor will rely on effort to manipulate dramatic action instead of relying on preparation and process. Yet, by forcing emotion to happen in a certain way, the actor creates tensions that lodge in the musculature and end up blocking emotion.

When the actor stops creating these tensions, the feeling may well come up of its own accord and seek external expression. When the actor's process works well, intention leads to action through the imagination alone. The actors really listen to each other, hear each other, and respond to each other; neither is caught up in judging what just happened, nor is in the throes of anticipating what will happen next.

For this to take place, though, the actor has to overcome stress, or, rather, react differently to it. Stress has two components: the stressor, and the individual's response to the stressor. The actor cannot change the stressor (the special characteristics of the theatrical situation), but he can manage his response to the situation. Physical and psychological changes occur in response to stress, generating a heightened physical and mental state. This is normal and desirable, for it improves performance. But sometimes the changes are not so welcome; if overwhelmed by stress, the actor will tighten his neck, grip his back, raise his shoulders, brace his chest, and stiffen his limbs, while his heartbeat races and his temperature fluctuates. These are not the responses of the character but of the actor, and the actor needs to use all his skill not to let this heightened state of tension interfere with the behaviour of the character.

The Alexander Technique can play a vital function by helping the actor manage his or her self-created tension thanks to inhibition and direction. Through awareness of what is happening to himself (or, more precisely, what he is doing to himself), the prevention of inappropriate automatic habits of use, and the redirection of his neuromuscular system, the actor organizes his good use and attains poise, co-ordination, freedom, and openness to the moment. Engaging in this process, it is possible for the actor to maintain perspective on what is happening and not to become unduly anxious or tense.

As the pressure rises in rehearsal and performance, the stimulus to tense up and interfere with the process is greater. In moments of high emotion on stage, it is particularly important to work within a free instrument. The actor needs to remain released as an actor while fully engaged as a character, if he expects to perform well repeatedly over time. John Harrell, actor and MFA graduate of SMU, faced this difficulty playing Orgon in a very physical production of *Tartuffe*:

> The rage was an important part of the character, who lashed out against a world that just would not listen to him or take him seriously. However, I out of necessity had to construct a physical shell that was as relaxed as possible and yet still seethed to the audience. If I allowed the emotion to create the posture by itself, it ripped apart my back. Many times I would sense that my body temperature was far too high and therefore I must be working too hard. I learned to have the actor's thought process while using the Alexander process to inhibit and then make the best possible choice in the moment.

Sometimes the demands of a rôle and the overt appearance of good use dovetail harmoniously. A well co-ordinated character allows the actor to be well co-ordinated too, in a manner that does not draw undue attention. At other times, a rôle may require that the actor inhabit a body with alien physical characteristics: a hump or a limp, a hangover, arthritis, paralysis, for example. An actor who plays a character with potentially disabling misuse must organize the character's co-ordination with mental attention, not muscle tension.

The Alexander concept of use can provide a key to the character's body, to what is possible and necessary, to what feels and looks right. What is this character's postural behaviour? How does he hold his spine? How does he walk or gesticulate? Suppose the character misuses himself. I can explore how to inhabit a tense body without making myself unduly tense. I do not need to be destructively tense for the audience to get the message of tension – any more than I need to be pathologically mad for the audience to witness madness. My character slouches, but I lengthen and widen within that slouch, remaining as open as possible within the constraints set by the choice of physical characterization. The challenge is to perform the appearance of misuse repeatedly over time without harm and without getting stuck in the reality of misuse.

I coached a production of *One Flew Over the Cuckoo's Nest*, which required many cast members to wrestle with this problem. The inmates of the asylum at the heart of the play manifest their unique psychological disturbances through idiosyncratic patterns of misuse and distortion. One actor whose character hallucinated chose to be almost doubled over, tailbone tucked under, chest collapsed, head poking forward, eyes intensely open. By lengthening, widening, and releasing within these attitudes, the actor could continue to breathe and not stiffen, and could walk away performance after performance without any pain. The actor moved consciously into the appearance of misuse from his own best use, explored the nature of misuse, and consciously moved out of misuse.

My student Jo Benincasa faced a similar situation when he performed in Sam Shepard's *A Lie of the Mind*.

I had to play a character who, among other things, gets shot through the leg and rots away on a couch. At a particular moment on stage, I had to become very upset and raise my voice considerably, all the while remaining helpless on the couch with my leg propped up. I was having much trouble getting into the emotion of the moment, because I was unable to use my body to rant and rave (the actor's easy cop-out when expressing anger). Instead, I over-used and misused my voice, relying solely on my throat to carry the scene.

With a lot of coaching, I was able to do two things: first, to focus on the words of the scene and what I was trying to communicate; and second, to continue to release my head and neck and allow the breath in and out as was natural to the moment.

This part of the performance became very technical for me, and I was constantly falling out of the moment in order to focus on releasing and breathing, and on the target words I had shaped to convey my message. My voice was free and the lines were clear, yet I was still unable to let go and just do it.

In a tech rehearsal, my scene partner and I were forced to go over the scene four or five times for a light cue. We had to be stopped every time, as I lost touch with the moment. A while later, Chad and I were joking around during the breaks in which the lights were being adjusted. When we went back to the scene, I lazily let my awareness go and I just did the scene, all the while expecting to be stopped as before. To my surprise we did the whole scene without a hitch. Having technically scripted out the vocal and physical patterns of the scene, and after letting go and having a good laugh, I was now freely reacting to my fellow actor, completely immersed in the moment; and the performance elevated itself from technical to truthful. I had made a breakthrough. Awareness does not have to be forced, and good use is not always conscious.

With training, the actor may become aware of himself without becoming self-conscious. The actor can learn not to over-work physically, not to mis-direct effort or attention, and not to let adrenalin or anxiety derail the performance. The double process of inhibition and direction is operative even when adrenalin and anxiety are both at the highest possible levels, as attested by my student Jodi Benker:

This past June I went to camp in Seattle, where for three weeks I trained to become a stuntwoman. The training was vigorous and challenging. It consisted of hand-to-hand combat, armed combat, trampoline work, falls, stunt and precision driving, work on horseback, high falls, fire burns, snare and jerk harness work, squib work (with guns and windows), and rock climbing. Needless to say, it was a very packed and strenuous three weeks.

I had recently completed a year's study of the Alexander Technique. Those lessons saved my back or neck from being broken one day at camp, when we were doing horseback work. Besides riding the horses, we had to make them do all kinds of sideways walking, come to sudden stops where we almost went flying off the front of them, and – the kicker – we had to fall off at full-speed gallop! Of course you did not have to do it if you did not want to, but I am a sucker for trying anything once. I had to fall off this horse named Sassy, looking like I had been shot and being all dramatic. This last ended up being easy, because I was truly terrified out of my mind. I finally got the hang of Sassy, sped up to a full gallop, and came up next to a mat of three feet by three feet – acres of room to hit at high speeds off the back of a horse, right? Well, it looked more like a speck to me. I prepared myself and removed my left foot out of the stirrup. Everything was going as planned, but when I threw all my body weight over Sassy to take a perfectly calculated hit at that mat, I swung down and hung off the side of Sassy like a worm on a hook. My right foot was supposed to slide out of the stirrup, but it did not budge. I was hanging in the air, twisted, one foot caught in the stirrup, half-off a galloping horse.

In a frenzy of panic, I told myself that if I used myself correctly I would get out of this situation with my back and neck still intact. I remembered to direct my body up and think my energy out through the top of my head. Before I knew it, I was slowly sliding out of the stirrup as Sassy galloped along the rail. I landed perfectly aligned on my back in the dirt.

Aside from getting all dirty, pointed at, and double-dared to do it again, I was fine. And, yes, I got up and did the whole thing again, because a good stuntwoman is the one that gets up to go to work the next day in one piece.

I am amazed by what our bodies can do with just one thought! All I did was think 'energy out and up', and I saved myself from being kicked, trampled or flattened. I made it through the rest of the camp and had a glorious time.

The actor can learn to create a physicality that contributes to the character without harming the actor. He or she can learn to be open to the moment, to be spontaneous, to be simple, and even to fall upwards off a horse. When an actor no longer creates tension and resistance in order to work, then he or she is simply free to go about the business of the character. This freedom is exciting. Thanks to it, the play or the film comes to life moment by moment, drawing in the other essential participant in performance – the audience – to connect with the truth happening in front of their eyes.

CHAPTER 9
The Teacher

THE EDUCATION OF A TEACHER – PATRICIA BOULAY

I started taking lessons in the Alexander Technique seventeen years ago, when I was a student in a dance school. At the time I did not suffer from physical problems, and my main reason for studying the Technique was to improve my understanding, as a dancer, of the workings of the body.

The Technique was from the outset a great revelation. It was evident to me that the questions I asked myself – about movement, balance, the economy of means in positioning the body – found clear, simple, and extremely precise answers. These came to me not intellectually or verbally, but, rather, through experience and sensation. Each Alexander lesson helped me understand the workings of my whole person. In that sense, the answers I received went well beyond my expectations. I had begun a journey of true self-discovery.

In my dancerly vision, which still separated the physical and the mental, I had at first perceived the Technique as a series of steps towards a greater awareness of my body. Instead, it turned out to be a profound undertaking meant to integrate the whole person. The interactions of all that is physical, mental, and emotional revealed themselves to me in their full intensity. I was opening my eyes, and – brought back to myself, to the here and now – I had to face my fears, anxieties, and blocks.

For me, the rebalancing of our propriocep-tion is one of Alexander's great discoveries. He found that the accumulation of tensions ended up deforming our sensations. The body becomes anaesthetized and we stop feeling its tensions and hindrances – in effect, we start navigating with a false compass. If we do not sense ourselves any more, how can we listen to our hearts, our bodies, and our minds? Indeed, to rediscover harmony and health, we need to tune in to ourselves and re-establish the accuracy of our proprioception, which in turn changes our view of ourselves and of reality.

What is particularly remarkable about the Alexander Technique is the absence of physical exercises. Instead, you must seek to integrate its principles to daily life through a change in your manner of thinking and doing – whether in an ordinary gesture such as walking, sitting, or standing, or in a more complex skill such as playing an instrument or singing at a concert.

I left each Alexander lesson full of enthusiasm and nourished for the whole week. The more I progressed, the more the Technique interested me. Two years after the start of my lessons, I moved to England to pursue a three-year training course in the Technique. My motivation at the time was not to teach others, but rather to work more intensely on my own use. It seems to me that many people who choose to train as Alexander teachers share this motivation.

The training is above all practical, and consists in cultivating what Alexander called

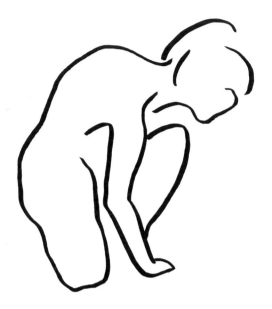

pupil by touch and through verbal guidance. The future teacher cultivates a certain inner calm, thanks to which she becomes able to listen to others. This quality of empathic listening allows the teacher to perceive and evaluate a pupil quickly and in great depth. The teacher then tunes herself to the pupil to work with him. Transmitting to the pupil her own inner calm, the teacher leads the pupil to listen to himself and to develop his sensitivity, attention, responsiveness, and openness. As the pupil finds his centre, which he strives to keep in his every activity, he becomes better capable of establishing this quality of empathic listening between him and the world around him, thus setting in motion a chain reaction.

My years of training were rich and difficult. In fact, the training is very much more than a simple 'technical' learning. For three years one undergoes great changes, with all the crises and doubts (as well as the euphoria and

'good use of the self', and maintaining this good use in order to transmit a new experience to someone else. There are no exams in the traditional sense, but a constant evaluation. The training is extremely demanding; in most schools it takes place three hours daily, every day of the week over three school years.

The Technique is taught in over thirty countries. In London, where Alexander spent most of his working life, there are hundreds of certified teachers and at least half a dozen training schools. I chose to attend the training course directed by Patrick Macdonald, who had taken his first lessons as a child from Alexander himself, and who had trained as a teacher in the early 1930s. Mr Macdonald was a demanding man, yet sensitive and full of humour. Recognized as one of the leading lights of the Alexander profession, he attracted students and teachers from all over the world. He died in 1991, aged 81.

The student who follows a training course must create and renew a state, a way of being, which she then learns how to transmit to a

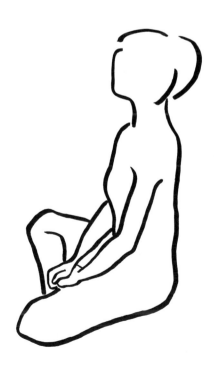

enthusiasm) that profound change always entails. Needless to say, during my training I applied the Technique to my dancing; I derived intense pleasure from my new-found ease, fluidity, and lightness, although, with time, dancing receded into the background and the Technique itself became the centre of my life.

Teaching the Technique has allowed me to deepen and refine the paradoxes of Alexander's principles; I grew to understand that the conscious will must work to stop, to master, and not to act – for, when we act, the body becomes an object and takes on a mechanical function, which hampers action. Conscious will is evidently needed, as are desire and goal-setting, yet it is important to know the limits of volition. The well-directed will, imbued with patience and listening, derives its strength from a constant exchange between thought and feeling.

(Patricia Boulay teaches the Alexander Technique in Vincennes, near Paris, France.)

HOW TO FIND A TEACHER

Throughout this book, men and women who have studied the Alexander Technique have shared their experiences with you. You have also met Alexander teachers from several backgrounds – a Brazilian musician, an American woman of the theatre, a Canadian runner, a French teacher and mother. You now have an understanding of the principles of the Technique and of its applications to many fields. It is perhaps reasonable to expect you to be convinced of the merits of our work, and to be ready to take lessons in the Technique. Now you need to find a good teacher.

In 1958, three years after Alexander's death, a group of teachers trained by Alexander formed the Society of Teachers of the Alexander Technique (STAT). STAT aims to maintain and improve professional standards, encourage research in the Technique, and prevent abuse and exploitation by untrained people. All teaching members of STAT have completed a full-time, three-year training course, and hold comprehensive insurance. Members are bound by a Code of Professional Conduct.

STAT organizes an annual conference and a memorial lecture. It publishes a newsletter three times a year and a scholarly journal at irregular intervals. Anyone interested in supporting the aims of STAT may become an associate member and receive its materials.

At present there are teachers in more than thirty countries all over the world. Several countries have their own national societies, which are affiliated to STAT and share similar professional standards; below you will find the addresses of all the affiliated societies in English-speaking countries. STAT will provide you with a list of teachers and affiliated societies worldwide.

STAT
1st Floor, Linton House
39–51 Highgate Road
London NW5 1RS
Phone +44 (0)845 230 7828
Fax +44 (0)20 7482 5435
www.stat.org.uk

In the United States, please contact:
AmSAT
PO Box 60008
Florence, MA 01062
Phone: +1 (800) 473 0620 or
+ 1 (413) 584 2359
Fax: +1 (413) 584 3097
www.amsat.ws

In Canada, please contact:
CANSTAT
RPO 984 West Broadway
PO Box 53568
Vancouver, BC V5Z 1K0
Phone: +1 (877) 598 8879
Fax: +1 (604) 879 3744
www.canstat.ca

In Australia, please contact:
AUSTAT Inc
PO BOX 716
Darlinghurst, NSW 2010
www.alexandertechnique.org.au

In South Africa, please contact:
SASTAT
39A Arnold St
Observatory 7925
Cape Town
Phone +27 (21) 448 5514
www.alexandertechnique.org.za

There are teachers and training courses outside STAT. Some of these are grouped into professional organizations, of which the largest is called Alexander Technique International (ATI). Their web site is on www.ati-net.com

Evaluating a professional in any given field is always complex. How does one find a good stockbroker, a good mechanic, or a good dentist? Judging an Alexander teacher is perhaps even more difficult, since the Technique – based on *non*-doing – is likely to resemble nothing that you have encountered before. At first, you may not fully understand or appreciate what the teacher is trying to do. In other words, you may need to have quite a bit of experience in the Technique before you are able to tell whether or not a teacher suits you. (Of course, this also applies to dentists and stockbrokers, and to all the other professionals with whom you must deal.)

We all tend to measure and judge others according to criteria that are not necessarily practical or useful. A teacher may be charming and pleasant, but incompetent; it would be preferable to study with an insightful teacher even if he or she has a difficult temperament. It is also possible for a young and newly trained teacher to have better discernment than a seasoned professional who has embraced dubious ideas. In brief, it is preferable to choose competence over charm, and talent over notoriety. If you ever find a teacher who is charming, talented, competent *and* experienced, count yourself privileged and share him or her with everybody you know.

If there are no teachers in your area, bring together a group of like-minded people and invite a teacher to come and give a series of conferences, workshops and lessons. STAT or your national society will publish your invitation in its newsletter.

TEACHING YOURSELF THE TECHNIQUE

If it is really impractical (due to distance, for example) for you to take lessons from a certified teacher, it is not impossible to learn the Technique without the help of a teacher. After all, Alexander did it himself, but you should remember that he was a man whose creativity, perseverance, and capacity for observation – among many other attributes – were all extraordinary. For us, men and women of average ability, the task is infinitely more arduous. If you do decide to study the Technique alone, you may wish to consider the following observations about the principles of the Technique.

- The Alexander Technique is not a method of working on your body, for there is no separation between the physical and the mental. In every situation, every part of your entire being plays a constructive role. Good use entails an attitude as much as the co-ordination of the whole body.

- The Technique is not a method of relaxation. Rather, it seeks to cultivate right tension – right in quality and amount, in the right places, for the right length of time. Relaxation is a side-effect of right tension.
- In the Technique you do not learn to do the *right* thing. Rather, you learn to *stop* *doing* the wrong thing, and the right thing does itself.
- The means determine the ends directly, and the ends determine the means indirectly. If you use the wrong means, you have no hope of achieving your ends.
- Keep in mind at all times that there may be – there almost certainly is – a gap between what you think you are doing and what you are in fact doing.

Good luck.

CHAPTER 10
Conclusion

'NEVER HEARD OF IT'

I had never heard of the Alexander Technique before reading your book, and yet I consider myself well informed.

Alexander started teaching his Technique more than a century ago, and opened his first training school for teachers in 1930. STAT, the first professional body grouping trained Alexander teachers, was founded in 1958, and today there are nearly 2,000 teachers world-wide. Despite its long history and its fundamental contribution to the fields of education, medicine, sport, and the arts, the Alexander Technique remains relatively unknown outside a few circles.

The term 'Alexander Technique' works against us. The word 'Technique' implies to some a mechanical approach to mechanical problems; although the Technique is eminently practical, there is nothing mechanical about it. In addition, calling it by the name of its founder (thereby paying rightful homage to a great man) personalizes the Technique to a certain degree (thereby dimming its universal character). Imagine how different the history of psychoanalysis would have been if it were known as 'the Freud Technique'.

Several aspects of the Technique make it difficult to explain and to make it known. The Technique redefines a number of concepts – relating to the body, the mind, tension, relaxation, posture – in such a way that only somebody who has had practical experience in the Technique may apprehend these new definitions without equivocation. Language stands in the way of intellectual understanding. I say 'tension', and I mean one thing; you hear 'tension', and you understand something else. However, if you were to take a series of lessons with me, you would come to share, through experience, my practical definition of the word. Then we could talk about the Technique and understand each other.

The American philosopher and educator John Dewey, known as one of the two foremost exponents of pragmatism (the other being William James), was greatly influenced by Alexander. He had many lessons in the Technique and wrote introductions to three of Alexander's books. In one of them, Dewey states that 'the principle and procedure set forth by Mr Alexander are crucially needed at present. Strangely, this is the very reason why they are hard to understand and accept.' They are needed because faulty sensory awareness makes us end-gain and misuse ourselves; and they are hard to understand and accept precisely because of our faulty sensory awareness, which Dewey called 'this perverted consciousness which we bring with us to the reading and comprehension of Mr Alexander's pages'.[45] Because of the ever-pervasive phenomenon of faulty sensory awareness, the Alexander Technique is not suited for work in large groups (*see* Chapter 4). It is difficult therefore to expose enough members of the public to the Technique to achieve a critical mass of recognition and acceptance. Although private lessons in ballroom dance and in Italian may well be more useful than group classes, those subjects (and many others), as traditionally taught, allow ten, twenty or more people to learn at the same time. The Technique, however, must be learned individually, and over a long period of time, which makes its growth slow and laborious.

In my opinion, efforts to make the Technique better known and more widely accepted have been based on flawed assumptions. There are teachers who see the Technique as part of the larger, so-called New Age movement, yet it belongs squarely in the mainstream of contemporary thought. Placing it aside from the mainstream does the Technique a disservice. Other teachers have been keen to conduct scientific studies in the Technique, in the hope of explaining or proving its physiological soundness. While this may in principle help some people embrace the Technique more readily, it also risks doing the Technique more harm than good. Psychology may give us some insight into why people end-gain, while physiology may perhaps explain how people misuse themselves. In a sense, though, psychology and physiology become one in the Technique, and lose their pertinence as a result. You end-gain; because you end-gain you misuse yourself; because you misuse yourself you suffer; if you inhibit and direct, you can stop end-gaining, misusing yourself, and suffering. The point can be so easily demonstrated that it is irrefutable. Writing about some of the problems of modern medicine, Dr Oliver Sacks points out that 'a split [has] occurred, into a soulless neurology and a bodiless psychology'.[46] By its very nature, the Technique is able to heal this split, and attempts to deconstruct it physiologically and psychologically may be a step backwards, not forwards.

Most people today look for easy, short-term solutions to their problems, preferably ones that will not demand effort or responsibility. We take drugs with the sole purpose of suppressing symptoms of disease, when a real cure would require sacrifices, such as changes in lifestyle, giving up alcohol or cigarettes, or the slow and steady cultivation of character. We consult astrologers hoping to hear that the source of our problems lies in the stars. (This is not to dismiss astrology, which, when intelligently practised, may be a good source of information about individuality.) Most people who first seek out the Technique often have an unstated attitude towards their teacher: 'Take care of me.' The teacher's attitude is just as simple: 'I can only teach you to take care of yourself.' One extraordinary thing has happened to me several times over the years: at the end of a lesson, the pupil takes out a diary to write in the next appointment, and, instead of writing 'Alexander lesson,' or the name of the teacher, finds herself writing down her own name. It is a revealing lapse of the pen; during the 30 or 40 minutes of the lesson the pupil is truly taking care of herself.

The Technique demonstrates constantly that our problems are inseparable from our beliefs and our behaviours, and that their solution entails self-awareness, personal responsibility, and the control or elimination of many habits that please us, despite their detrimental effects on our health. Inhibition, however, does not come naturally to everyone. Even when the Technique offers excellent, durable, and cost-effective solutions to their problems, pupils sometimes prefer to go elsewhere, having found the demands of self-awareness too daunting. I think many teachers have had the experience of giving fine lessons to new pupils who run away once they come to the realization that well-being is a choice that they must make for themselves daily, all day long. As William James once said, we must get out of bed in the morning looking for good health. Lying on a table and allowing an Alexander teacher to lengthen and widen you is delicious. Having to lengthen and widen by choice in the face of life's constant challenges is another matter.

Although the Alexander Technique is built on timeless principles, it is not wholly in tune with the mood of the times. Current mores are based on self-expression; the essence of the Technique is self-restraint. As I argued in Chapter 5, in the long run self-restraint leads to greater personal and professional fulfilment than self-indulgence. The difficulties of learning how to inhibit make the goal unattractive to some in the short term. Still, if by inhibiting you become free, strong, focused, independent, healthy, and possibly even happy, then one day you will, like me and many others, be thankful for Alexander and his genius.

'WHAT IS THE ALEXANDER TECHNIQUE?'

Augustine once said, 'What is time? If you do not ask me, I know; if you ask me, I do not know.' I started studying the Alexander Technique in 1978, and I have been a certified teacher since 1986. I spent seven years preparing my first book, *Indirect Procedures*, before embarking on two versions of this, my second book about the Technique. Yet I have never found a good answer to the simple question: 'What is the Alexander Technique?' My only comfort is that my difficulty in giving a precise, elegant, and unequivocal answer to this question is shared by everybody who has ever travelled the Alexander route.

Nobody should ever assume that the words he or she uses in a given conversation are used or understood in the same manner by other participants in the dialogue. Certain terms that are perfectly clear to the initiated – the self, inhibition, direction, use, functioning, the Primary Control – are not at all useful in

a brief exposé directed to a total beginner, as their connotations in fields unrelated to the Technique make it difficult for the novice to grasp their meaning.

Some of the concepts of the Technique negate the clichés of received wisdom, and listeners are confused, and sometimes put off, when their beliefs are challenged. When he saw a gesture that seemed to him to be well executed, my teacher, the late Patrick Macdonald, would exclaim with pleasure, 'Lots of lovely tension!' It may be difficult to believe that there is such a thing as lovely tension (the tension needed for this or that gesture, which is appropriate for this or that situation). All the same, the Alexander Technique is frequently dismissed as just another method of 'physical relaxation'. Did I say 'physical'? There is no separation between the body and the mind, or between all that is called 'physical' and all that is called 'mental'. Indeed, Alexander did his best to avoid using the word 'body', both in his teaching and in his writings. Perhaps you understand why, if you followed my arguments throughout the book. Yet, how is it possible to convince somebody that all that he does – including his every thought, his every breath – show to the world the wholeness of his being? How can we stop him taking care of his 'body' at some point of the day or the week, and looking after his 'mind' at a different time? Medicine tells him to do this; his entire education, from childhood onwards, has led him to think in that way, and language itself makes it difficult to behave differently. Tension, relaxation, posture, physical health, mental health, intelligence, will, spontaneity, freedom – each of these words stands for a more or less absurd abstraction.

If I could have you in my hands, make you react to a situation that differs from those you encounter habitually, make you lose your balance a bit, and make you come out of your cocoon for a little while, you would see that your whole being is present in everything that you do. You would see how your reactions are automatic and outside your conscious awareness. You would notice, perhaps for the first time, that you do too much, too soon, too awkwardly. After a series of practical experiences, you would finally understand that you end-gain, and because you end-gain you misuse yourself, and because you misuse yourself you suffer. You would realize that the difficulties of daily life – what you call 'stress' – are not caused by others, but, rather, by your way of seeing others. Little by little, you would start inhibiting your normal reactions and directing your Primary Control, as well as the rest of yourself. Little by little, you would stop *doing* and *blocking*, and you would start *allowing* instead, thereby arriving at a truly natural state. In short, if I could have you in my hands for a while, I would give you a practical demonstration of the Alexander Technique, showing you something that I will never be able to explain in written paragraphs.

'You will notice,' wrote Mr Macdonald, 'that those who know little about the Technique often talk and write more about it than those with greater experience of it.'[47] Beloved master, I shall say no more.

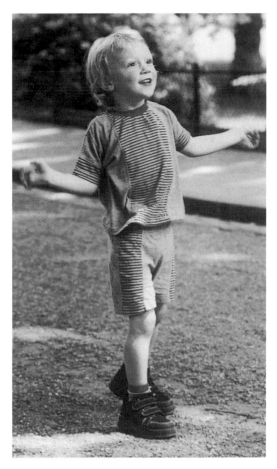

Bibliographical Notes

1 'Ethology and Stress Disease,' in *More Talk of Alexander*, ed. Wilfred Barlow (London: Victor Gollancz, 1978), 250.

2 *The Use of the Self* (Kent: Integral Press, 1955; first published in 1932), 1.

3 *Articles and Lectures* (London: Mouritz, 1995), 207.

4 *The Use of the Self*, 27.

5 'Appreciation', in *The Universal Constant in Living* (Long Beach (CA): Centerline Press, 1986; facsimile of the 1st (1942) ed.), p. xxi.

6 *The Art of Piano Playing*, trans. K. A. Leibovitch (London: Barrie and Jenkins, 1973), 101.

7 *Articles and Lectures*, 203.

8 'Training with F. M.,' *The Alexander Journal* 12 (Autumn 1992): 28.

9 *Man's Supreme Inheritance* (Kent: Integral Press, 1957; first published in 1910), 188.

10 *Constructive Conscious Control of the Individual* (Downing (CA): Centerline Press, 1985; facsimile of the 1st (1923) ed.), 201.

11 Quoted in Sir Charles Sherrington, *The Integrative Action of the Nervous System*, 2nd ed. (New Haven: Yale University Press, 1947, 1961), 259.

12 Sandra Blakeslee, 'The Physical Roots of Emotion,' *International Herald Tribune*, 8 December 1994, 8.

13 *Labyrinths: Selected Stories and Other Writings*, ed. by Donald A. Yates and James E. Irby, with a foreword by André Maurois (London: Penguin Books Ltd., 1970), 276.

14 *Constructive Conscious Control of the Individual*, 146.

15 *Articles and Lectures*, 206.

16 Ibid.

17 Quoted in Perry Garfinkel, 'Beat Stress All Day,' *Men's Health,* January/February 1997, 84.

18 *Articles and Lectures*, 203.

19 *The Alexander Principle* (London: Victor Gollancz Ltd, 1991), 129.

20 *Articles and Lectures*, 204.

21 Ibid., 139.

22 2nd ed., rev. Sir Ernest Groves (Oxford: The Clarendon Press, 1968), 295.

23 'Ethology and Stress Disease,' 254.

24 Ibid., 252.

25 Ibid., 254.

26 *Man's Supreme Inheritance*, 167.

27 *Running with Style* (Mt. View (CA): World Publications, 1975), 4.

28 *The Universal Constant in Living*, 106.

29 In Richard Williams, 'Age of the Rocket Man,' *The Independent on Sunday Review*, 20 June 1993, 11.

30 Quoted by Alexander, *The Universal Constant in Living*, 110.

31 *Running with Style*, 36.

32 *Athletics: How To Become A Champion* (London: The Sportsman Book Club, 1961), 87.

33 *Constructive Conscious Control of the Individual*, 291.

34 'From 7th Stringer to 7th Heaven', by Lowell Cohnn, *International Herald Tribune*, 15 December 1997, 19. All quotes

about Montana are from this article.

[35] *The Art of Piano Playing*, 109.

[36] *International Herald Tribune*, 23 October 1996, 20.

[37] *International Herald Tribune*, 31 October 1996, 19.

[38] *The Universal Constant in Living*, 216.

[39] *The Integrative Action of the Nervous System*, p. xvi.

[40] 'Appreciation,' in *The Universal Constant in Living*, p. xxviii.

[41] Quoted in *The Art of Piano Playing*, 33.

[42] Ibid., 32.

[43] *Notebooks 1924-1954*, trans. Shaun Whiteside, ed. and with an Introduction by Michael Tanner (London: Quartet Books, 1989), 9.

[44] *The Art of Piano Playing*, 79.

[45] *Constructive Conscious Control of the Individual*, pp. xxi, xxii.

[46] *The Man who Mistook his Wife for a Hat and Other Clinical Tales* (New York: Harper Perennial, 1990), 93.

[47] *The Alexander Technique as I See It* (Brighton: Rahula Books, 1989), 25.

Further Reading

Learning the Alexander Technique is no different from learning how to sing, in that taking lessons from a good teacher is perhaps the only way of progressing well. Reading cannot replace the practical experiences, but may well enhance them. The bibliography of the Alexander Technique grows steadily every year. In the United States, AmSAT (www.amsat.ws) offers a book service with a large selection of books, articles, brochures, and audio and video tapes on the Technique and related subjects. In the United Kingdom, the publisher Mouritz (www.mouritz.co.uk) specializes in books about the Alexander Technique. It ships its own titles, as well as a selection of books by other publishers, worldwide. The following list is far from exhaustive, and is meant to help you get started on your further reading.

Alexander wrote four works, which are intermittently in print in various British and American editions. There exist a fifth volume, of collected articles and letters, and a sixth book, of summaries of Alexander's books by a journalist who knew Alexander. Alexander's writing style is very much of his own time, and modern readers sometimes find his books difficult to grasp and digest. However, they are full of insightful arguments and telling anecdotes, and a disciplined reader should find them a source of enlightenment.

The Use of the Self, Alexander's third book, is perhaps the most accessible for a beginner pupil to read. A slim volume, it contains Alexander's own account of how he discovered his technique (which, as I mentioned in the first chapter, Nikolaas Tinbergen declared 'one of the true epics of medical research and practice'), two case histories (of a stutterer, and of a golfer who could not keep his eyes on the ball), and chapters on use, reaction, and medical diagnosis.

At the time of writing, these are the available editions of Alexander's books:

Man's Supreme Inheritance (London: Mouritz, 1996) (first published in 1910)
Constructive Conscious Control of the Individual (London: Mouritz, 2004) (first published in 1923)
The Use of the Self (London: Orion Books, 2001) (first published in 1932)
The Universal Constant in Living (London: Mouritz, 2000) (first published in 1941)
Articles and Lectures (London: Mouritz, 1995)
Ron Brown, *Authorized Summaries of F. M. Alexander's Four Books* (London: STAT-Books, 1992)

For a well-written and informative history of the Technique, together with biographical information on Alexander, his brother A. R., and the men and women who played a role in developing the Technique, *see* Frank Pierce Jones, *Freedom to Change* (London: Mouritz, 1997).

For a doctor's view of the Technique, *see* Wilfred Barlow, *The Alexander Principle* (London: Victor Gollancz, 1990).

For a thorough study of the Technique applied to a sport, *see The Art of Swimming*, by Steven Shaw and Armand D'Angour (Bath: Ashgrove Press, 1996); and *The Art of Running*, by Malcolm Balk and Andrew Shields (Bath: Ashgrove Press, 2000).

For a study of the applications of the Technique to pregnancy and childbirth, *see The Alexander Technique Birth Book*, by Ilana Machover, Angela Drake, and Jonathan Drake (London: Victor Gollancz, 1995).

The most comprehensive study of the Technique and the performing arts is my book, *Indirect Procedures: A Musician's Guide to the Alexander Technique* (Oxford: Clarendon Press, 1997).

My website contains book excerpts, original articles and essays, and links to other sites of interest: www.pedrodealcantara.com

Index